(handwritten) Clause Hitchison '91

Scapegoats

Scapegoats are a universal phenomenon, appearing in all societies at all times in groups large and small, in public and private organisations. Hardly a week passes without some media reference to someone or something being made a scapegoat. Tom Douglas examines the process of scapegoating from the perspectives of victims and perpetrators, tracing its development from earliest times as a rite of atonement to the modern forms of the avoidance of blame and the victimisation of innocents. The differences and similarities between the ancient and modern forms are examined to reveal that despite the modern logical explanations of behaviour, the mystical element in the form of superstition is still evident.

The theories and explanations which social scientists have evolved to define scapegoating as a form of social behaviour are examined and the processes of its management and resolution are covered in detail. Finally, Douglas analyses the distinction between the 'rational' form, i.e. the deliberate and intentional victimisation of innocents in order to ensure personal survival, and the 'irrational' form, i.e. the response to frustration of unknown or wrongly attributed causes.

Scapegoats will be an invaluable resource for all professionals engaging in groupwork and groupworkers in training.

Tom Douglas has over forty years' experience of working with groups and for many years worked as a freelance groupwork consultant.

Scapegoats

Transferring Blame

Tom Douglas

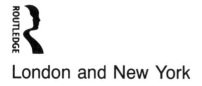

London and New York

First published 1995
by Routledge
11 New Fetter Lane, London EC4P 4EE

Simultaneously published in the USA and Canada
by Routledge
29 West 35th Street, New York, NY 10001

© 1995 Tom Douglas

Phototypeset in Times by
Intype, London

Printed and bound in Great Britain by
TJ Press (Padstow) Ltd, Padstow, Cornwall

British Library Cataloguing in Publication Data
A catalogue record for this book is available from the
British Library

Library of Congress Cataloguing in Publication Data
A catalogue record for this book has been requested

ISBN 0–415–11018–1 (hbk)
ISBN 0–415–11019–X (pbk)

**To Shirley with love as ever,
for her patience and support.**

Contents

Part I

Ancient ritual

The ancient process of the transfer and disposal of evil, which has come to be known as 'scapegoating', seems to have existed ever since human beings held the concept that they were under the supervision of divine beings. However, it is a moot point which arose first: the perception of divine beings or the human's wish to be absolved from culpability, to escape punishment, to stop a process of entailed consequences. Whatever the truth may be, it is certain that Tyndale's development and use of the word 'scapegoat' provided an accurate and easily understood means of describing a process that is extremely basic to the human condition.

The three chapters in Part I are concerned with the origins of the term and with a description of the ancient processes of scapegoating. The aim is to define the purposes and consequences of the performance of these rituals and to consider the role of those selected to be victims whether inanimate, animal or human.

Chapter 1

Origins
Tyndale's word and its continued use

Scapegoat – Any material object, animal, bird or person on whom the bad luck, diseases, misfortunes and sins of an individual or group are symbolically placed, and which is then turned loose, driven off with stones, cast into a river or the sea, etc., in the belief that it takes away with it all the evils placed upon it.

(Maria Leach 1950)

In 1590 Robert Kers was stricken with a disease which was believed to have been laid upon him by a warlock while he was at Dumfries. Agnes Sampson, a witch, cured him by taking the disease upon herself and then attempted to transfer the disease to either a cat or a dog, by means of laying cloths upon these animals. However, Alexander Douglas of Dalkeith apparently touched the cloths before the animals and as a result wasted away and died. Agnes Sampson was later convicted of witchcraft. This story, recorded by Frazer,[1] describes very clearly another major aspect of the scapegoating procedure, the belief that evils, disease, bad feeling, etc., can be transferred from one person or object to another by the performance of the appropriate rituals. Of course, the fact that the poor soul who caught the disease and died was a member of the family of Douglas adds a certain piquancy to the tale for me.

Dr George Habash, a leader of the Popular Front for the Liberation of Palestine, was allowed into France at the end of January 1992, ostensibly to seek treatment in a Paris hospital after having had a stroke. Habash, described as a terrorist and a man wanted by the Israeli government, was admitted to France while President Mitterrand and his Foreign minister were on a state visit to Oman.

The outcry which this event caused was predictable and, as a result, French Interior Ministry Officials resigned, as did the head of the French Red Cross responsible for flying Dr Habash into the country. *The Daily Telegraph* described the situation as 'a decision mind-boggling for its political ineptitude and moral impropriety'.

At this time President Mitterrand's government was recorded as becoming increasingly unpopular, with the prime minister Mme Edith Cresson reported to be deeply unpopular and lacking in authority over her ministers.

What was done was wrong, without doubt, and as a consequence people were punished, as was to be expected. But lying behind the justice of such punishment was a very considerable feeling that had the government been more popular the resignations and sackings would have been regarded as excessive. What justification is there, then, for such a response?

Because the government was seen as weak it was attacked with more ferocity than previously. Thus, in order to stay in power with some semblance of authority, the government had to overreact to assuage the wrath of the population. This was done by sacrificing very publicly people who were important enough to satisfy the public but who may have had little or nothing to do with the original scandal. They were in effect the *scapegoats*. The blame was attached to them and they were despatched to the political wilderness.

Seldom does a week pass without some reference in the media to someone who has been made a scapegoat. Indeed, it would not be stretching the truth to say that it has become one of the favourite words of the latter half of the twentieth century to describe those in public, and in private, who are apparently unjustly or unfairly blamed for certain events.

ORGIN OF INTEREST

I have been fascinated by the idea of the scapegoat ever since, as a small boy, I encountered the term in readings at Sunday School. For many years this fascination was more or less dormant and was only occasionally sparked into life by references in the press, on the radio and in conversation about people and groups who were deemed to have become, or been made, scapegoats by others. Then, as my interest in painting and art history was aroused, I came across Holman Hunt's painting of the scapegoat.

When I started to work with groups of people it became obvious that scapegoating was a ubiquitous occurrence in groups of all sizes. Now the term started to be surrounded and complicated by ideas like blame, prejudice, visible difference, intense dislike, frustration, displacement and maintenance. I watched members of groups being made scapegoats and worked hard to try to understand what was happening as well as to try to learn how to prevent the apparently harmful manifestations that occurred.

I was now intrigued by what was seemingly ancient ritual behaviour in modern groups. Was there, or is there, an aspect of human behaviour that is universal and manifests itself in attempts to diminish or alleviate guilt and fear of punishment by some form of transfer of responsibility onto someone or something else? Where does the concept of the tangible nature of 'bad' originate, enabling it to be redirected like a stream of water or a current of energy from one human being to another or to some other living creature and even to inanimate objects? Can this transfer be effected by a simple ritual pattern? What level of belief must exist about the nature of things – and about the process of the accumulation of 'badness' in particular – to consider that such a method of dispersal might be effective? Do the current psychological and sociological approaches by attempting to be logical and rational miss something which is part of the mainstream of human experience? If so – what?

Is there some basic need in human beings to ward off responsibility, to transfer badness to others even though, currently, we would eschew the ritual and mystical aspect of such an idea? But from whom or what do modern blame-shifters seek to evade censure? Someone has to take the blame to allow the rest of us to continue our normal functions, nominally at least, free of guilt or responsibility for events past.

Within the therapeutic milieu of groups, groupwork and group therapy – and also within organisations – people are often referred to as 'scapegoats' and reference is frequently made to the process of scapegoating. Within groupwork much has been written about the act of scapegoating – the process of being a scapegoat – and a very distinct and well-defined concept or series of concepts has emerged. In essence these tend to put the scapegoat as a person who is, in some ways, necessary; by taking the responsibility of blame for some of the bad things that are happening to the group and within the group, a scapegoat can make it possible for the group to continue to function. Consideration must also be given to the method by which the scapegoat is chosen by the group or organisation and to the way in which some scapegoats select themselves.

In this respect, the element of victimisation is very great, but the entire concept of the scapegoat – i.e. a person standing-in for others in order to accept blame and responsibility for some occurrence – is as old as humanity itself.

It is my intention to trace the behaviour patterns that were established around the scapegoat concept, blame-laying and blame-acceptance and maintenance, and to follow their development and change through the ages to the modern usage.

Mary Renault,[2] in her book *The Praise Singer*, gives a graphic description of a scapegoating process from ancient Greece (see quotation at the head of Chapter 2).

As we shall see later, people like this victim were selected because they were malefactors or diseased and were often stored and maintained by the city until such time as they were needed to fulfil their role, which inevitably ended in death.

ORIGINS OF THE WORD

William Tyndale, born in Gloucester in 1494, scholar and protestant, translator of the Bible, was strangled and burnt at the stake by the Catholic establishment at Vilvoorde a few kilometres north of Brussels in the year 1536. After his death his prophecy, that he would have made it possible for a ploughboy to know more scripture than the scholars, started to come true. Indeed, when the English translation of the Bible was undertaken after 1538 it was based essentially upon Tyndale's translation, but in order to prevent an outcry the translation was credited to one Thomas Matthew.

In this way Tyndale's version of the Bible survived through King Henry's Great Bible, and a great deal of it is still to be found in the King James Bible, the authorised version.

Tyndale's reading of Leviticus, chapter 16 verse 10, is as follows:

But the goat, on which the lot fell to be scapegoat, shall be presented alone[3] before the Lord, to make an atonement with him and to let him go for a scapegoat into the wilderness.

And verses 21–2 offer:

And Aaron shall lay his hands upon the head of the live goat, and confess over him all the iniquities of the children of Israel, and all their transgressions in all their sins, putting them upon the head of the goat and shall send him away into the wilderness by the hand of a man who is in readiness. The goat shall bear all their iniquities upon him to a solitary land; and he shall let the goat go into the wilderness.

It is generally accepted that Tyndale invented the word 'scapegoat' to express what he understood to be the literal meaning of the Hebrew word 'azazel', a word which appears to have several meanings. For instance, Milton[4] says that Azazel is the standard bearer of the rebel angels. In Mohammedan demonology, according to Brewer,[5] Azazel is the counterpart of the devil, having been cast out of heaven for a refusal to worship Adam. His name is then rendered as Eblis (Iblis), which means despair.

Yet again, Azazel as a being appears as a vicious wilderness demon similar to Lilith the vampire demon. Then the man who was deputed to take the goat into the wilderness in the Hebrew atonement ceremony, usually a person regarded as being disposable and often unclean, was customarily identified with the animal. In the passage of time, any kind of unfortunate outcast came to be known as Azazel.

Another form of the word 'Azal', this time used as a verb, has the meaning of 'to remove'. In its reduplicated form of Azazel it was occasionally used to emphasise the meaning, e.g. to remove completely.

Given these complexities of possible meanings, from where did Tyndale derive the word 'scapegoat'? In order to discover this we shall need to look rather more closely at the ritual that the passage in Leviticus was describing.

Brewer[5] says about this ceremony that it was

Part of the ancient ritual among the Hebrews for the Day of Atonement laid down by Mosaic Law ... two goats were brought to the altar of the Tabernacle and the high priest cast lots, one for the Lord and the other for Azazel. The Lord's goat was sacrificed, the other was the scapegoat; and the high priest having, by confession, transferred his own sins and the sins of the people to it, was taken to the wilderness and suffered to *escape.*

The italics are mine, and have been used to bring into prominence the word 'escape'. Most authorities, when writing about the scapegoat of the Day of Atonement, actually describe the goat as being 'driven' into the wilderness. If Tyndale had read into the Hebrew the idea that the goat was 'suffered to escape', then his coining of the word 'scape' goat becomes much clearer.

The word 'scape' is what the dictionary describes as an 'aphetic' form of the common word escape, i.e. it has lost its first letter and was a form used in the thirteenth century. *The Oxford Dictionary of English Etymology*[6] records that Tyndale 'intended to render the supposed literal meaning of the Hebrew Azazel... "the goote on which the lotte fell to scape" '. This translation led in turn to the Vulgate using the phrase 'caper emissarius' and to the French translation becoming '*bouc emissaire*'. The dictionary goes on to suggest that the correct interpretation may well be 'a goat for Azazel' who, as we have already seen, was a wilderness demon. Now this raises an interesting question. The Bible expressly forbids the worship of demons (Leviticus 17.7) and yet we are being told that if the first goat was for the Lord then the second goat was for Azazel, he being a demon.

The only other prevalent use of the aphetic form of escape appears to be as 'scapegrace', which also carries a religious connotation in that a person so described was one who had *escaped* the grace of God. This manner of use was prevalent in the nineteenth century, having replaced the earlier version of 'wantgrace'.

The word 'scapegoat' does not appear in later translations of the Bible. For instance, the Revised edition of 1884 inserts the name Azazel and has a marginal note which offers 'dismissal' as an alternative reading.

It becomes fairly clear that what Tyndale was trying to convey by the use of the word scapegoat was a significant difference between the process of sacrifice, which was the fate of the Lord's goat, and that of the ritual transfer of evil. In the second process, death might be the ultimate outcome as far as the scapegoat was concerned. Indeed, as we shall see many times and in different places, it was the intended outcome, but it was certainly not the prime reason for the performance of the ritual.

Indubitably this was to cleanse the community of its sins by the process of transferring the sins to an animal and allowing it to escape into the wilderness. The fact that the animal could be in contact with others or with human beings, and that the sins might then transfer to them, seems to have been a matter of little concern. Indeed, in later versions of this ritual of transfer of evil there is obvious and deliberate intent to transfer it to others irrespective of whether this contact will bring about their death or diseased state.

The process of transfer we shall take up at length later. However, as we are here concerned with the word itself, it may be of interest to note that there are two other words in the English language which have the connotation of the transfer of evil or of misfortune. The first and perhaps older of the two is 'sin-eaters'. They were people who were employed by relatives of the dead to take upon themselves the sins of the dead person by the process of eating beside the corpse. Essentially this process was deemed to deliver the soul of the deceased from having to spend time in Purgatory.

Brewer[7] describes a particular example of this ritual as follows:

> In Carmarthenshire the sin-eater used to rest a plate of salt on the breast of the deceased and place a piece of bread on the salt. After saying an incantation over the bread it was consumed by the sin-eater and with it he ate the sins of the dead.

The very clear perception demonstrated by the relatives of the dead person – that it was possible and desirable to transfer the sins of the deceased to another who, presumably, would then have to bear those sins unless others could be found to bear them instead – is close to the concept of the transfer of sins that took place in the ritual of the scapegoat, the major difference being that it was a ceremony performed for the already dead in the case of the sin-eater but for the living in the case of the scapegoat. Also, the ceremony was performed for the benefit of one person rather than for a community, but we shall discuss this in more detail later.

The other English reference to the transfer of evil or bad feeling occurs in the words 'whipping boy'. The element of transfer becomes subtly merged with the idea of substitution, for the whipping boy was a young or inferior person whose duty was to accept punishment for wrong-doing performed by his or her superior.

When royal persons were deemed to be ruling by divine right and to be in some senses gods themselves, the idea of physically punishing one of them in their early years for misdeeds was unthinkable. But, nevertheless, the punishment demanded either by the manner of upbringing or by law had to be administered. Thus, substitutes were found who received the punishment, whatever it was, on behalf of the erring prince. The act of substitution runs parallel with the concepts of transfer as we shall see, but the modern use of the word scapegoat often confuses these concepts and the term is used indiscriminately. When we look at other modern terms we find that those like 'fall guy' and 'dupe' and the processes of 'framing' and 'setting-up' have a much stronger connotation of cynical exploitation for personal security than of ritual transfer. The major reason for this may lie in the enormous difference in the belief systems of the communities involved.

Tyndale's invented word has a long history of use, but there is one final point to be made before we start to look at the reasons for the behaviour it was coined to describe. This is the problem of anachronistic use.

This section has been titled the 'origins of the word' for the simple reason that Tyndale's word has been used quite naturally to describe forms of behaviour that are similar to the atonement rituals it first stood for, but because it seems to have been so effective it has also been used to describe similar rituals that existed long before Tyndale. There is, of course, nothing intrinsically wrong with this; it is often difficult to find words adequate to describe complex behavioural patterns, and when one is discovered which does the job well by being easily and accurately understood, it is used with vigour.

There is, however, the problem that a superficial likeness used to describe situations hundreds if not thousands of years apart can diminish real understanding of the differences. In my case the similarities are important because they may lead to a discovery that there exists an area of human behaviour which, although superficially similar, is also essentially similar at a much deeper level although the communities in which that behaviour occurs have changed considerably.

Because I have had an interest in the processes and outcomes of scapegoating for a great number of years both from an historical view point and from the practical necessity of having to deal with the process when faced with it in various group situations, the references and quotations I have used cover a span of some forty years. Those I have used here have been selected in preference to others on two very important criteria. First, they illustrate the changing attitudes to the process of scapegoating over those forty years and, second, they seem to me to illustrate most clearly what I want to convey. The latest commentaries are not invariably the best nor the most apt. As Karl Popper once said, 'There can be no reasonable ground for believing that a new theory contains more truth than the old.'

One further point should be made: although I have reason to believe that scapegoating is a worldwide phenomenon, my experience has been confined to western Europe and I have therefore drawn most of my historical development sequence from material on western culture.

NOTES

1 The story of Agnes Sampson occurs in Frazer's discussion of the transference of evil. He says, 'The notion that we can transfer our guilt and suffering to some other being who will bear them for us is familiar to the savage mind. It arises from a very obvious confusion between the physical and the mental, between the material and the immaterial' (p. 166).

2 In Mary Renault's story the citizens of Ephesus were threatened by the army of the Medes, so they selected as a sacrificial scapegoat, a swindler. Renault describes the problem of choice between two possible victims and also the hate that was transferred to the selected victim because of the fear inspired by the approach of a barbarian army.

3 Sometimes given as 'alive'.

4 In *Paradise Lost* (p. 534) Milton, describing Satan rallying his legions, portrays Azazel as the standard bearer.

> 'Then strait commands that at the warlike sound
> of trumpets loud and clarions be upreard
> His mighty standard; that proud honour claim'd
> Azazel as his right, a Cherube tall:
> Who forthwith from the glittering staff unfurl'd
> Th' Imperial Ensign, . . .'

5 Brewer has several points of interest, for instance:

'In Mohammedan demonology Azazel is the counterpart of the devil, cast out of HEAVEN for refusing to worship ADAM. His name was changed to EBLIS (Iblis) which means "despair".' He became the father of devils (p. 62).

'SCAPEGOAT. Part of the ancient ritual among the Hebrews for the day of ATONEMENT laid down by Mosaic Law (see Lev. xvi) was as follows: two goats were brought to the altar of the TABER-NACLE and the high priest cast lots, one for the Lord, and the other for AZAZEL. The Lord's goat was sacrificed, the other was the scapegoat; and the high priest having, by confession, transferred his own sins and the sins of the people to it, it was taken to the wilderness and suffered to escape' (p. 967).

Day of Atonement or Day of Coverings was the '10th day of the first month, Tishri. It is observed by a strict fast and ceremonies of supplication, the whole day being spent in prayer and confession' (p. 1172).

6 The etymological dictionary states that probably the correct interpretation of scapegoat should be 'a goat for Azazel', the wilderness demon. This would seem to suggest that Tyndale intended to render the supposed literal meaning of the Hebrew Azazel.

7 Brewer places great stress upon the fact that sin-eaters were hired; taking on board the sins of another was a business transaction.

Chapter 2

Purification and propitiation
Scapegoating founded in the belief systems of society

They stripped him, and put the ritual offering cake in his hands, having to tie them there, because he shook so, and led him out to the gate. There they beat him as the rite prescribes, on his tenderest parts till he screamed aloud. Then everyone fell on him as they chose, to purge their offences which he carried for them, and drove him along with sticks and cudgels till he fell. I don't know if he was dead when they came to throw him on the bonfire.

(Mary Renault 1979: 40)

The victim in this incident described by Mary Renault was known as the Pharmakos (Φαρμᾱκός) which is defined in Liddell and Scott's *Lexicon* (1896: 752) as 'one who is sacrificed as a purification for others, a scapegoat: then since worthless fellows were reserved for this fate, an arrant rascal, polluted wretch'.

Indeed, the victim described in *The Praise Singer* was a polluted wretch in the eyes of his society and we shall consider how victims were selected in detail in the next chapter. Of more immediate interest is our concern to look at the process that has been labelled 'scapegoating' – that is, at the activities, motives and interests of those who initiate the ritual. Immediately two factors stand out clearly, both well illustrated in the incident quoted above.

As we have seen (Chapter 1), the Greeks sacrificed their pharmakos because they were afraid of the approaching army of barbarians at whose hands there must have been some expectation that they would suffer, if not be killed. Implicit in this expectation is the belief that nothing of even the smallest moment could occur without it being the will of the gods and with their involvement directly or indirectly in bringing about events. Then it was only logical that some approach should be made to the gods to ameliorate the potentially damaging events that were about to occur or to change or halt them. Thus a process of pleading, of offering gifts, was most obviously the path that could be followed.

This process encapsulates a great deal of what we must examine more closely in the actual process of scapegoating but, first, it highlights the element of fear as the propelling motivation to seek for ways of allaying imminent peril and, second, it shows that the process of propitiation was a communal effort. The whole society was in jeopardy from an invading army of barbarians, in this instance Medes; the gods were the 'supervisors' of that society – and supposedly of all others – and, therefore, the whole community took an active part in the process of appeasement.

The scapegoat ritual was essentially a process of purification, which means in essence that its practitioners felt that they were contaminated by the transgressions of their daily lives and that the ritual of scapegoating was one that would effectively disperse that contamination and reinstate them as clean in their own eyes and, more importantly, in the eyes of their god. The three basic elements of this process can be made quite clear and the all-encompassing element must be the belief system in which the ritual was practised.

The ancient Hebrews believed in a divine being who was all powerful, all seeing and able to reward and punish at will. The nature of that belief is of little moment but the consequences of holding it are absolutely essential to any understanding of the scapegoating process. The Hebrews believed that their god had created what could be called a set of rules by which life was to be led, which included strict observance of prescribed rites, the performance of rituals of worship and a moral code. Whoever failed in the observance of these rites was deemed to have transgressed a divine code of behaviour and was thus held to have sinned. Sinners were bound to be punished because one of the attributes of the divine being was to be able to know everything, no matter how trivial, that took place. This factor of total observation, the first of the three basic elements mentioned above, has then to be correlated to another essential fact of the belief system, which was the human being's inevitable proclivity to sin. This led directly to the prospect of punishment, which, due to the omniscience of the divine being, was inescapable. The inevitability of punishment coupled to an obvious human trait to attempt to avoid hurt could only be achieved if a channel of communication to the god was established and could be used.

Escape from punishment for transgressions could not be expected to be granted without some cost to the suppliant or the sanctions against transgressing would be seriously enfeebled. Thus it was necessary to have some form of penance which would involve cost in order to earn the forgiveness of the god.

Without some concept of supervision by an all-powerful being with the perceived ability to punish wrong-doing, no development of the rituals of purification and propitiation would ever have taken place. This fact, stated here in such a bald form, becomes very important later when we consider what or who is being propitiated in modern scapegoating processes. Perhaps we may be faced with the idea that the ritual of the scapegoat in an extremely distinct religious culture was really an overt expression of some innate behaviour of human beings designed to reduce psychological discomfort and practically in terms of self preservation.

The second essential element, stemming from the acknowledged frailty and tendency of human beings to transgress, is the need for constant repetitions of the process of supplication for forgiveness. This ensures that, in the case of the Hebrew scapegoat, it became an annual event which, as Graves (1961: 195)[1] points out, occurred usually at the beginning of the agricultural year and in his opinion was inextricably linked to rituals for ensuring a successful harvest. But, certainly, repetition which must have stemmed from urgent need originally would ensure eventually that the whole process became ritualised and its essential meaning standardised.

The third and most important fact of the belief system which was ritualised in the scapegoat procedure was the idea that evil, sin and badness all possessed some form of substantial existence, which meant that it could be handled in appropriate ways and thus transferred to and from inanimate objects, animals and humans. Of course, this involved a set form of ritual; as we shall see, words and ritual actions were regarded as able to effect change – they were instruments of power. Thus it was that the sins of a community could be ceremonially laid upon the selected goat and the animal driven or led out into the wilderness. The sins of the community thus being removed like the disposal of rubbish.

An essential fact of this exercise, as the name 'scapegoat' given by Tyndale implies, was that the animal was allowed to escape. As long as the goat departed from the boundaries of the community, carrying with it all their wickednesses, it was left to wander as it willed. The fact that it may not survive was not an essential point. Nor, given their deep belief in the transferability of evil, was the fact that in its progress the goat might come in contact with other animals and humans and could inflict the sin-burden it was bearing onto them. They may have believed that such an event could not occur without the appropriate words of power being involved, but later generations of scapegoats had no such belief and it was understood that sins could be transferred from the scapegoat to whoever or whatever came in contact with it. It may be pertinent to note in this instance that the scapegoat was believed by the Hebrews to be carrying its burden of sins into the domain of the wilderness demon Azazel, which would seem to indicate that they were actually returning sins to those beings whom they believed were responsible for encouraging the sinning behaviour of man in the first place.

Whatever the reality of this procedure it is certain that both the Hebrews and their deity were able to accept (a) that purification and cleansing had taken place on its completion and (b) that the need to punish had been avoided. The justifiable anger of the god at human inability to live a righteous life had been assuaged and life could be resumed without the prospect of immediate and devastating punishment.

BELIEF SYSTEMS

Let us now examine some of these factors of the belief system in which scapegoating arose so that later developments in the process, culminating in modern practice, can be compared with them to ascertain the changes that have taken place over the centuries and the elements that have remained the same.

Writing about the power of myth, Campbell (1972: 22) said:

And if one should ask why or how any such insubstantial impulsion ever should have become dominant in the ordering of physical life, the answer is that in this wonderful human brain of ours there has dawned a realisation unknown to the other primates. It is that of the individual, conscious of himself as such, and aware that he, and all that he cares for, will one day die.

Campbell then defined the three great impulses in mythology, which were, first, humanity's recognition of its own mortality; second, the recognition that his society pre-existed each individual's appearance in the world and would continue after he had gone; and, third, the individual's gradual awareness of his or her power of thought and of observation of what was going on all around.

> Myths were not devised simply to entertain and amuse, but to explain things – to account for reality.
>
> (Baigent *et al.* 1986: 158)

Part of the belief systems of the ancients which appears in many places and among many peoples is that their gods were responsible for creating the world out of chaos and that the process of establishing order is a continuous process which, if abandoned, would automatically permit chaos to reassert complete sway in the universe.

> At the Creation God mounted the primordial hill. Out of Chaos he created Order, binding Himself and His Creations by law which henceforth would sustain that order. Thereafter it was violated only at great peril. If a king governed without due regard for truth and justice, the land would be scourged by plague, famine and foreign invasion.
>
> (Tolstoy 1985: 217)

Whether gods were invented by men to meet their needs and hopes, as Feuerbach believed, or men were created by gods is of no significance. What are important are: (a) the existence of a belief system in a particular society; (b) the strength with which it was held or enforced; (c) the extent of its distribution through the population; and (d) the effect it had on behaviour patterns. In other words, we are here concerned with consequences, not causes.

For instance, if a society believes that not only did their gods create the world in which human beings live, including the humans themselves, but that the whole of this massive creation is dependent for its continued existence upon the maintenance of the goodwill of these selfsame gods and that human beings have a major role in this maintenance system, then it is only logical that they should also believe that disobedience could result in the end of their world and also that nothing could conceivably happen without the sanction of the gods or their express intervention. As Tolstoy implies in the above quotation, contravention of the gods' wishes by important human beings would result in punishment. The ultimate punishment which the prescribed activities of humans kept at bay was the restoration of absolute chaos.

The belief systems of the ancients also included a perception that all things were linked, so that what we would call inanimate objects had some form of life and attributes – and all natural things likewise. Thus the world and all the spaces around the world were full of invisible entities, spirits and forces, many of which were inimical to human beings while others were generally benign, but all of them capable of some form of intervention in human affairs and all of them supposedly susceptible to bribery and placation.

> Following from the concept of wyrd was a vision of the universe, from the gods to the underworld, as being connected by an enormous all-reaching system of fibres rather like a three-dimensional spider's web. Everything was connected by strands of fibre to the all-encompassing web. Any event, anywhere, resulted in reverberations and repercussions throughout the web.
>
> (Bates 1983: 12)

This interconnectedness described by Bates is part of a pre-Christian belief and is not so different in some of its aspects from the ideas of the modern chaos theorists. What tended to spring from such belief were rituals involving sacrifice which were intended to maintain the very essentials of life. For instance, the Aztecs believed that the sun would not rise each morning unless offered the blood and hearts of sacrificed humans.

> By the time the Spaniards arrived the ceremonial year had become a grisly round of human sacrifice. Children were drowned to please the rain god. Women danced in the temple

knowing that their heads would be slashed off as they did so. Prisoners were flayed so that priests could dress up in their skins. And above all there was the insatiable thirst of the sun.

(Gascoigne 1980: 185)

From this idea of a belief system we can isolate several factors which have some fundamental bearing on the process of scape-goating. They can be enumerated as follows:

1. The idea of supervision – the omniscient, omnipresent god.
2. The fallibility and frailty of human beings.
3. The expectation of punishment.
4. The idea that humans can communicate with gods.
5. The need for atonement, penance and repentance.
6. The fear of failure and the need for repetition of propitiation.
7. The acceptance of the transferability of evil.

There are also three other factors we must consider briefly, which are not so clearly linked to the belief system *per se* but are essentially part of the scapegoating process:

8. Fear and ignorance of the causation of natural events.
9. The idea that the bearer of evil was not killed as sacrifice.
10. The act of scapegoating was performed as a communal ritual.

Supervision

One of the major elements of the belief systems of the ancients is the perception that all human beings are totally exposed both in thought and action to their gods. This has the principal effect of inspiring mortals with a sense of guilt, well aware that in everyday life they constantly behave and think in contravention of the rules laid down by their gods, provoked in such behaviour and such thoughts by personality factors and their responses to situations.

Guilt is an extremely uncomfortable emotion and it is not surprising that methods of discharging its power were well estab-lished very early in humanity's relationship with gods. We shall consider these methods later but it must be stressed here that even monotheistic societies believed that the supervisory process of the god was ably carried out by such divine minions as angels and other spirit beings.

The belief that an all-seeing god is aware of everything that an individual does in even his or her most private and secret moments has to lead to a feeling of considerable awe and a great degree of fear. Therefore, several ways of coping developed, among which was a belief that the all-seeing god was not only infinitely wise but also just in that transgressions would not be punished in an unfair and biased way. The process of defining god in this way could lead to his being personified as a loving father, strict, but caring for his children, whose main aim was to ensure their care and development. In this process people could then believe that punishment administered by their god was for their own benefit.

Another form of dealing with the idea of consistent and all-pervading supervision, whether for human benefit or not, was to create some form of acceptable appeasement. This commonly took the form of an offering of some kind. It is interesting to note that traditionally the gods were offered the thing that was most precious to human beings – that is, the food upon which survival depended, or life in some form, which was frequently the life of a human being.

The third method of dealing with divine supervision, and the recognition that all transgressions would be recorded, was to devise a process by which human beings would admit their sins and then go through a ritual of cleansing to rid themselves of their offences in the sight of god. This method, as we shall see later, was dependent upon a perception that transgressions, sins, evil, disease, illness, etc., possessed a tangible and transferable existence.

Thus it is possible to differentiate between two different kinds of sacrificial offering in the scapegoating procedure which are certainly confused by some commentators. The 'tributary' offering, which would normally be a gift to the god for his personal use, in essence a goodwill gift, was designed to maintain good relationships with the god or to prepare the way for later requests for favours. In some sense this form of sacrifice is designed to alter the balance of obligation somewhat in favour of the less powerful figures involved.

The second type of sacrifice was 'piacular', which was expiatory in character and design, brought about by the need to expiate some offence or to avert some potential evil or disaster in the sense of the pharmakos referred to earlier. It is into this type of sacrifice that the scapegoat appears to fit in the sense that the offender(s) is basically the sacrifice, having forfeited his or her life to atone for some sins. A substitute, however, was usually found unless the real offender was actually an offender against the civil law as well as a transgressor against holy writ, in which case that person's life was really forfeit.

When we consider in the next chapter those who became victims in the classical scapegoating procedure, it will be noted that those who had offended against civil law and been found guilty were often those selected as substitutes for others whose failing was sinful rather than criminal – a case of good economic practice in the use of scarce resources when both kinds of sacrifice could be fulfilled in the one process by the use of a life already deemed expendable.

The fallibility of human beings

Even a cursory survey of the early books of the Bible reveals an astounding number of detailed laws governing all aspects of behaviour and the kind of punishments, both human and divine, which transgression entails. Granted, as scholars have suggested, large numbers of prescriptions and prohibitions relate to the society and the nature of the land in which it was based. Without doubt such a detailed mass of laws indicate that this was a society in which its members found it more than difficult to live strictly within the bounds they had been set.

All human failings are listed in the books of Moses clearly in anticipation, if not in knowledge, that such failings were going to occur in abundance. Here are transgressions of holy law and civil offences side by side. This leads to the speculation that if such fallibility was expected and prepared for in terms of the prescribed punishments, then there would also be prepared methods by which repentance and expiation could be used. Human emotions, ambitions, aggression, avarice, love, hate, etc., provide the motivation for behaviour that is not only self-seeking but also contrary to both civil and holy law.

Behind all this lies the inevitable fact of mortality which must have made most ancient peoples aware that they had only a short period of mortal existence which, given their fallibility and their inclination to sin, was one they would seek to preserve and even to prolong. Thus offerings which could assuage the divine wrath, and penance which could prevent severe punishments of a physical kind that would diminish not only the quality of life however meagre, but in many cases its extent, would certainly be regarded with great favour.

The same preoccupation with the sins and crimes of humanity can be seen just as readily in the Koran. For instance, p. 379: 'As for those on the left hand (wretched shall be those on the left hand) they shall dwell amongst scorching winds and seething water: in the shade of pitch black smoke, neither cool nor refreshing', which is one of the milder threats of punishment to come for those who do not live according to the strict codes of behaviour.

All of which leads directly to a consideration of the rewards for good behaviour, a life among the blessed after death and the punishments for bad behaviour.

The expectation of punishment

> Garments of fire have been prepared for the unbelievers. Scalding water shall be poured over their heads, melting their skins and that which is in their bellies. They shall be lashed with rods of iron.
>
> (Koran, translated by N.J. Dawood 1990: 236)

Early societies seem to have believed that the most effective way to keep a society functioning was through a system of rewards and punishments technically based upon the judgement of one or more divine beings. Both the Old Testament and the Koran are stocked with admonitions to good behaviour, with rewards clearly specified and the punishments for infringement outlined with judicial detail. The essential fact about this is not so much that such a reward/punishment system existed but the consequence of believing that it did. This presents us with the problem of trying to determine whether a basic characteristic of human beings has always been a strong urge to evade, as far as possible, the more serious consequences of some kinds of behaviour.

For survival human beings have had to develop skills, some of which are group based but others are clearly individualistic and self-preservative. When humanity recognised its own mortality however early that occurred, it is only logical that people would seek to preserve their lives as well as they could. That could take several forms, one of which would be to attempt to avoid situations that would be likely to terminate a person's existence or drastically to reduce its level of comfort. This would inevitably mean some attempt to avoid punishment, revenge or other life-threatening events. However, another way of prolonging but not preserving life would be to accept that death, in the right circumstances, would not be total extinction but entry into a new and better life.

The fear of punishment for wrong-doing on the one hand and the promise of the conquest of death on the other were powerful instruments for governing behaviour. For our purposes there is another consideration, which is quite simply that most human beings were driven by their natures and by circumstances into transgressing the approved codes of conduct. Given the powerful incentives just noted, it is very sensible that they should seek to find ways of obtaining forgiveness for their wrong-doing which would not completely obliterate their claim to a better life after death. Thus, because they could both forfeit this life and the next, and because humans are prone to be incapable of sustaining a totally sin free existence, it became necessary to have at least some form of negotiating possibility with the gods who were judges and arbiters and whose decisions were announced by their servants on earth, the priesthood.

Communication with the gods

There had to be at least one form of communication with these all-powerful, all-seeing, all-knowing beings and there also had to be some form of payment for wrong-doing which would serve to appease the wrath of these divine beings and stay their much feared punishments.

It is in this area of directly addressing the gods through personal supplication that some form of prayer develops. But there arises also the performance of rituals which tended to be supervised by priests who became the intermediaries acting between humanity and god and also there are the live and the inanimate representations of gods which can also be addressed directly.

The course of communication was always beset by the difficulty of attracting the attention of a god and also by the apparent fact that gods were more likely to pay attention to requests for forgiveness or anything else if they were offered some form of inducement. So it became necessary for supplicants to offer what was regarded as invaluable in their own existence, i.e. food, often burnt because smoke usually drifted upwards to where the gods were supposed to dwell and because it was thought to be assimilable in this form, which was as close to the non-corporeal state of the gods as humans could make.

Another problem in communication with the gods was quite simply the nature of the reply. Communication is a two-way process in which the sender has no real idea of whether he or she has succeeded until a response is received from the individual to whom the message was directed. Given the fact that gods tended to be, for the most part, invisible then any would-be communicators were dependent for the completion of the process on being told by those licensed to do so, i.e. the priests, that their messages had been received or by accepting some sign or symbol as providing an answer, or finally waiting to see what happened, believing implicitly that messages despatched in the approved manner would be heard but not necessarily acted upon.

As with all the factors we are considering here, the quintessential motivating basis is faith or belief. Thus, when societies started to become less afraid of their gods and endowed them with ever-increasing human characteristics, including emotions and a tendency to error, the belief in the ability to communicate actually increased but fear of punishment declined, as did the belief in the all-powerful nature of gods. So in Greek mythology we have the spectacle of gods fighting gods, taking sides in human conflict and also the sight of ordinary mortals decrying the wisdom and power of the gods and actually defying them.

The methods of communication with gods is essentially bound up with the nature of the belief system of a society which, in turn, is based upon their perception of the power the gods are able to invoke.

Penance, atonement and repentance

Thus in the traditional language of faith there was an injunction to 'repent for the Kingdom of God is at hand'. The idea was that because of human sinfulness a great catastrophe overhung humanity. God would come in judgment, and people must purify themselves and change their lives if they were to have any chance of surviving.

(Cuppitt 1985: 12)

Most of the ideas of penance, atonement and repentance have been covered earlier. It only remains to emphasise here that the need to seek forgiveness for sins and wrong-doing is based almost entirely on the need to secure survival both for the individual and the society in which he or she lives. Seeking forgiveness can only take place where the supplicant believes (a) that it is necessary for survival and (b) that the entity being petitioned is powerful enough to punish the impenitent wrong-doer and compassionate enough to forgive the transgressions of mortals if asked in the appropriate manner.

As the rabbis of the Roman period would say many centuries later, 'We have been taught that deeds make atonement for a man, and that repentance and good deeds are a shield against punishment.'

(Abba Eban 1984: 14)

More recently the quest for the reassertion of innocence was stated by Camus as being pursued at the cost of accusing everyone else, and even the gods if necessary. But whereas at present we protest innocence merely as a matter of our own defence and to preserve as far as possible our standing, even when we know that innocence is not a true claim, the ancients believed that innocence could actually be returned, that sins could not only be forgiven but that the stain of such wrong-doing could be wholly eradicated and the individuals returned to a state of purity in their own eyes, in the eyes of their society and in the eyes of their god.

Perhaps it is but a short step from achieving atonement and forgiveness by personal sacrifice to achieving the same result by the sacrifice of other things. For instance, in Leviticus we read that there were two goats: one, the scapegoat, was driven or led into the wilderness bearing the sins of the community; the other was killed as a sacrifice. It is not a great step from sacrificing a goat to sacrificing a human being, and many societies offered human sacrifice to achieve, as they thought, divine intervention on their behalf. What is quite interesting is that whereas the animals offered in propitiatory sacrifices could always be seen as representing high value to the society, the humans usually offered were frequently criminals and those of least worth.

Failure postponed and the need for repetition

If the processes of purification and propitiation were successful, then at the moment of completion of the ceremony, however performed, the individuals and community had what amounted to a clean slate and a fresh start. However, as might be expected, human beings have always had a considerable facility, over relatively short periods of time, of accumulating by their behaviour considerable quantities of evil, badness, disease, etc., and so the process had to be repeated.

Frazer (1978) noted this as the fear of failure. Essentially in early societies people were mortally afraid of crop failure and also of an inability to reproduce themselves. Thus Frazer believed that human scapegoats who were beaten to death were seen as embodiments of natural vegetation, the essentials of continued existence, and their sacrifice was 'intended primarily to refresh the powers of vegetation'.

Whether Frazer was right in his contention remains a matter for debate, but it is important to notice that the process of atoning for sins committed became an annual event, and in the case of the Hebrews it occurred at the beginning of the agricultural year. Why it was deemed expedient to allow sins to accumulate through a twelve-month period may otherwise be difficult to explain satisfactorily. There is, nevertheless, one factor of interest that is, in some degree, a contrast to modern practices of scapegoating; the ritual was a communal one. The whole population was involved to some extent and it is this fact that might have had some bearing on the restriction to an annual performance.

There is also the fact that the life cycle of plants was not believed to be a process of automatic renewal but one which required a great deal of effort on the part of human beings and gods to restart each year. The forces of chaos were ever present and order was something that had to be consciously and actively established and re-established.

Frazer believed that while a human scapegoat was used in the process of carrying away sins, if they were beaten and killed then their deaths were part of the process of ensuring the refreshment of the natural cycle.

The transferability of evil

> The transference of sickness and sin to a tree, animal or human being is a worldwide, usually annual, folk custom; it was practised in the ancient classical cultures and is common among all primitive peoples. In ancient Greece the scapegoat was often a volunteer, he was bedecked and led about the city, then stoned to death outside the walls.
>
> (Leach 1950: 976)

The transfer of evil is the basic premise of the scapegoat ceremony and it is one which, despite a growing awareness of what might be called scientific reality, has stuck with us in one form or another, debased though they may be, to the present day. We must therefore consider this phenomenon in some detail.

The modern understanding of the process tends to describe it as symbolic, and while that might satisfy current rational approaches, it seems to me to miss entirely the main patterns of the belief system of ancient peoples. Cuppitt (1985: 58) stated that words were not just the sounds of communication between human beings but were seen as being substantial forces in their own right. It was believed that certain words – pronounced at the right time, in the right way, and by the right person – could change and even instigate actual events, e.g. demons could be summoned, the weather influenced and so on. It is no great step, in a world in which everything was a manifestation of god, to believe that badness, evil, disease, etc., were entities that not only possessed a tangible if invisible presence but could be influenced by other factors such as words of power, incantations, etc.

Therefore, when the *Dictionary of Folklore, Mythology and Legend*, describing the scapegoating process, suggests that 'bad luck, diseases, misfortunes and sins' could be 'symbolically' placed on an object, animal or person, the prime point about the belief systems of ancient cultures who practised this form of ritual is somewhat minimised. Certainly substitution occurred insofar as one thing could be used in place of another, but there was no doubt that the reality of the process was of paramount importance. That is, when the words that transferred the evils the society wished to dispose of were said, then those evils were in fact transferred and the population cleansed. Such is the power of belief. The whole basis of the power of magic or witchcraft rests in the fact that those upon whom it is practised believe in the functional efficiency of the process.

Frazer (1978) suggested that this kind of belief was based upon a misunderstanding of the different nature of things and derived directly from the confusion between the mental and the physical, the material and the immaterial. Although we understand those differences today because our culture has had centuries of scientific enquiry to develop explanations of things and events, it is not to be countenanced that ancient societies were confused about such differences but simply that these societies did not question in the same way and sought answers in a totally different method of understanding.

Evils, sins, badness, diseases, bad luck and all kinds of misfortune were visited upon them by their gods, thus it would be acceptable to believe that if such things could be despatched to plague human beings, then it was logical that they could be diverted, passed on, dispensed with, in the same way. The gods by their actions of plaguing humans in fact demonstrated the transferable nature of evil. While human beings would not assume that they had powers equal to those of gods, the prevalence of ritual to transfer sickness and evil, whether onto others or not, throughout all early societies is sufficient reason to accept that humans devised various methods to divert such visitations.

It is not difficult to understand that where all inanimate objects had spirits, and where stones, trees, rocks, water could be concrete manifestations of supernatural entities, the transfer of evil and the efficacy of incantation and ritual would be as real as anything else in the world. It is important to realise that the sense of being able to influence events stayed with human beings through the use of such processes as cursing, casting spells, bewitching and enchanting and is still with us in the concepts of astrology, of bad vibrations and, of course, luck. Indeed, the bases of magic – of contagious magic and of imitative magic which Frazer considered to be the basis of the transfer of evil – are perhaps still with us in distorted and diluted forms.

Fear and ignorance of the causation of natural events

The basis of all ancient belief systems was fear. They, like us, needed to make some sense of the world in which they found themselves and there was much which seemed to be inexplicable unless it was deemed to occur under the auspices of forces they had no way of understanding or of controlling, and so much which rendered life a fairly perilous journey. If gods inspired fear, they could hopefully be appeased and thus their awesome power could be used at best to benefit humanity or at least its punishing and destructive nature could be diverted or diminished.

As we have noted earlier, all natural events including illness and death were understood only in terms of the decrees of gods. In modern terms the ancients stood in relation to their gods as powerless beings whose survival was wholly dependent upon total obedience, where the only ameliorating factor in the system was the process of propitiation.

The scapegoat was a messenger, not a sacrifice

The ancient Hebrews did sacrifice animals to their god and it is significant that the scapegoat was not killed. The animal had to leave the community alive so that it could take its burden of sin with it. Other societies killed their scapegoats, combining the functions of bearer of sins with that of sacrificial offering. Alternatively, by killing the scapegoat the sacrificers believed that the evil burden was also destroyed. However, as we shall see, many of these bearers who were killed were first driven clear of the community boundaries and often tossed onto waste ground when dead.

The idea of the scapegoat being allowed to live is of particular importance when we consider current practice, where victims are pushed to the periphery of a group or a community but not driven completely away because their function as a focus of blame may need to be repeated.

Scapegoating as a communal ritual

All that is needed here is to re-emphasise the fact that because the ritual of scapegoating occurred in relatively small populations numerically, and because the faith or belief system tended to be uniform throughout that population, the ceremony was a communal one. It was communal not just in the sense that every member of the community agreed with the procedure, but that they took an active part in it at the very least by being physically present and often, where beating was included, by active participation. Thus the whole community could feel it had cleansed itself.

The ancient Jewish belief system

The society in which the scapegoat of Leviticus existed had a belief system which combined most of the factors discussed in this chapter. To enumerate them, as did Cuppitt (1985:58), is in effect to summarise the chapter.

- Words were forces in their own right and could be used to modify events, create and alter situations and guide behaviour.
- Thinking was a process of deciding what to do on the basis of given ethical code.
- The idea of truth was contained in moral constancy and reliability.
- Knowledge was knowing the difference between what was right and what was wrong and being an obedient member of the community.
- Nothing about existence in the community was neutral – the whole of life was subsumed in the belief system.
- No theoretical knowledge existed in the belief system – all wants and people, all behaviour was enmeshed in the beliefs.
- Thus no explanations were available, just an acknowledgement that the world was as laid down in the scriptures and a complete obedience to the laws and devout allegiance was required.

'Knowing God is simply equated with doing righteousness.'

NOTE

1 Robert Graves suggests that Azazel was 'the scapegoat sacrificed by the Hebrews at the beginning of the agricultural year', thus making it a sacrifice to ensure a good harvest. He also comments that the 'scapegoat was a left-handed sacrifice' to Azazel, a manifestation of the goat Dionysos or Pan.

Chapter 3

Sin-eaters, whipping boys and fall guys
The role of 'victim' and the changes to it brought about by modifications of the belief system

Certainly the interpretation of human sacrifice suggested by Caesar is that the power of the gods could only be neutralised or controlled if one human life were exchanged for another. Thus if the Gauls were threatened by illness or battle, then the Druids organised human sacrifice, if criminals were not available, then the innocent would have to supply that life for a life.

(Miranda Green 1986: 28)

All through human history there have been ceremonies, if that is the right word, which have been and are described as scapegoating, and there have been victims. To place these events, rituals and behaviours under one common term must have certain implications which, baldly stated, can be limited to three for the sake of discussion. First, the term coined by Tyndale to describe a particular Jewish ritual of atonement defines an idea into which it is very convenient to slot a large variety of apparently similar behavioural patterns. Second, there is the possibility that although the term 'scapegoat' has been found convenient to describe religious and social behaviour occurring both before and after Tyndale's time, what it really defines is a remarkably consistent behavioural form. Third, there is the possibility that this remarkable similarity actually stems from the fact that behaviour described as scapegoating is the expression of a very deep human need.

It is obvious that these three implications are by no means mutually exclusive. Indeed, they may all exist at the same time so that we are faced with consistent patterns of human behaviour that are essentially conditioned by the belief systems of the societies in which they occur.

Understanding the way in which scapegoating takes form in different ages and societies is important, but so also is the nature of the explanations that are available to us of why it happens. This chapter will trace very briefly some of those differences, mainly marking the development of a rational and strategic use of the process of scapegoating, which is probably more individualistic than the ancient ritual but is equally dedicated to the purposes of evasion of responsibility or blame and to self-preservation. There is also a process of the transfer of blame, which is more a group phenomenon and appears to operate at a less conscious level. Its true nature is often unrecognised by those who operate it; indeed, who would tend to explain it in rational terms if asked, but whose rational observations are seldom rooted in objective fact.

Changes in society

The pattern of scapegoating over the ages appears to be dependent upon the kind of society or community in which it is performed and upon the prevailing belief system.

Perhaps the most significant changes in societies can be dealt with quite simply. Most obviously, communities have grown larger and have changed from agrarian to industrial; towns and cities have proliferated and have also grown much larger. As part of this growth people from different points of origin have been thrown together and are thus faced with different customs, habits and beliefs. This process has accelerated as large groups of people have taken up residence in a country that is not their country of origin and have brought with them even more different ways of living, beliefs, ideas, customs and behaviours.

The classic form of scapegoating took place in communities that were small in numbers and relatively homogeneous in their customs and belief systems. The process of scapegoating was a communal act of atonement, and while such communal scapegoating behaviour may still be found, the communal nature of the process is now mainly found in small distinct sections of the larger society, in parts of organisations and in small groups.

The main exception seems to occur when public figures are pilloried for their actions and they follow a procedure of selecting a scapegoat to take the blame in their stead. This rational/deflective process of scapegoating occurs because of the modern ease of communication. Ancient societies had little problem in communicating because city states, tribes, etc., were few enough in number to permit the most important activities to take place on a face-to-face basis. Modern societies have methods of communication that are as immediate as those early communal meetings, in addition to the immensely important factor of reaching a vastly greater number of people.

What has not changed in society is the simple fact of self-preservation, though it also seems to have become much more heavily weighted in terms of the survival of the individual, which tends to mean that communal loyalty is something that almost has to be created, nurtured and fostered. The most effective way of doing this in modern times seems to be by the appearance of some factor external to the society as a whole that could threaten every member without discrimination.

Throughout the ages it is possible to trace the continuous existence of a belief in the substantial nature of evil, badness and sickness and also of a belief in the ability to transfer them. There also continues to exist the belief that words have power in their own right and can influence events, and that there are supernatural powers who can and do interfere in human affairs – though the definition of such powers is far less clear than it once would have been and is much more related to individual tastes, beliefs and fears.

The gradual change in religious belief, mainly in its deterioration into superstition, is a factor of great importance, as is the development that some individuals were so important and necessary that it was deemed quite legitimate and indeed desirable that others should be punished in their stead for any wrongdoing. This concept of legitimate substitution plays a very important role through the times of such high status individuals as kings and emperors, dictators, individuals of power and wealth and other forms of great standing.

The belief persists that animals and inanimate objects could absorb evil and disperse it, and they are still used as objects possessing curative powers taking into themselves the evil and badness removed from human beings.

Finally there has been a great change over the centuries in two areas of human experience: first, in the area of moral standards and, second, in the enormous increase in the level of knowledge by the ordinary person. As we shall see later, the latter poses a great problem for although, through education and communication, the knowledge base of the average individual has continually expanded, this has been countered to a large extent by the astronomically huge expansion of the sum of knowledge that is now available. As a proportion of the knowledge available, it is debatable whether the ordinary individual actually knows more today than his ancestors. It is, however, important that each individual has come to regard explanation as possible and enquiry as necessary. Nevertheless, such great areas of ignorance that exist are still filled with beliefs which, while they may be much more personal than previously, are still beliefs and not rational knowledge.

Some of the major changes in all societies have occurred in their belief systems and it to those that we must now briefly turn.

CHANGES IN THE BELIEF SYSTEM

> When one begins to ask the question 'does it work?' or even 'does it pay?' instead of, 'is it God's will?', one gets a new set of answers, and one of the first of them is this: that to try to suppress opinions which one doesn't share is much less profitable than to tolerate them.
>
> (Clark 1971: 195)

The major changes in belief systems are those related to religious belief, but not wholly so.

The principal changes in the religious areas of belief have been brought about, first, by the proliferation of different religious faiths within individual societies and, second, by the tremendous move towards secularisation, particularly in western Europe. Counter to this has been the spread of religions and beliefs, originally of eastern origin, into the west and latterly the rise of extreme fundamentalism, mainly in Islam but also in other areas.

Cuppitt (1985) wrote that the process of secularisation saw a shift in the belief system from the position of 'explaining things by reference to occult powers', to a process of explaining them by 'reference to a built in law-abidingness'. This is a process in which religious and mythical explanations seem to be untrue, inessential and unnecessary. One factor which often appears to be overlooked, and is a consequence of increasing secularisation, is that the element of certainty which religion introduced into human existence – however spurious non-believers may regard it – has gone. Human beings have been faced with the loss of a prime support to their existence, which, given the fundamental terror that seems to be engendered by a contemplation of the total isolation of human existence, had to be replaced by some other form of certainty.

In essence this certainty has taken two main forms, one of which was to rationalise the religious belief by shredding away from it all the mystical elements while retaining the belief in a god. The second was to replace it by an acceptance of rational and scientific explanation.

As we noted earlier, the belief system of a society conditions the way in which the process of scapegoating emerges. However, the actual nature of that belief system is irrelevant but its consequences are vastly important. In the case of societies who are rapidly losing their traditional religious beliefs or being inundated with beliefs from other countries, the basic reason for the scapegoater's activities can be located in a different focus. If there is no longer a god or even supernatural or divine entities who supervise, reward and punish, who needs propitiating and who are susceptible to pleading and sacrifice, then to whom or to what is atonement directed in a secular, non-religious society?

This is both a simple and a very complex question. There are at least three main strands to a possible answer. Most importantly the process is directed at the society and community itself, and herein lies some of the complexity. The standards demanded of members of a society are deemed to be set by the society itself, but these standards are nowadays neither static nor wholly accepted. Tradition is a powerful setter of standards, but modern life tends to change so quickly that different parts of the same society, e.g. different age groups, may have very different standards and even very different beliefs. Thus the arbiter of an individual or group may be a small and distinct subsection of the larger community.

There are occasions when individuals and groups find themselves censured by the larger community, or at least by some very substantial part of it, and have need of some strategy to deflect and diminish that censure. In this event, the second area of concern – to whom is atonement directed? – provides the answer: it is the institutions of society that are able to highlight, publicise and expose behaviour and by so doing initiate censure, criticism and blame.

The third strand has to be approached with a degree of caution because it is fraught with complication. It is the individual's own sense of wrong-doing. The complexity lies in the definition, because although it may be described as conscience in one sense and therefore moral, it is just as likely to be an acute perception of what constitutes the bounds of public or community tolerance and of knowing the punishments and sanctions that are available.

Among those factors that are not replacements for divine supervision but are still part of the belief system we find the clear belief that most human events are susceptible of rational explanation. This leads ultimately to the stated belief that all interactive events involving individuals are caused by, encouraged by and acted out solely by individuals. Thus, when behavioural events occur which apparently have no rational explanation or even an obvious one, the implicit belief is that some individual or group is responsible. If no such individual or group can be located easily, some human agency is nevertheless held to be responsible. The factors that are paramount in deciding the human agency that will be selected to bear the responsibility of blame then become of supreme importance. Whoever is chosen, and how, the choice is still largely dictated by the belief system and by such factors as prejudice and difference, which we shall explore later.

VICTIMS THROUGH THE AGES

When human beings become the 'goats' in the scapegoating ceremony they appear almost universally to be chosen because they are different. 'Different' in this sense can mean that the chosen one is deficient in some obvious way, having some mark or some bodily defect. Frazer (1978) quotes instances in Uganda in which scapegoats actually had their legs broken after they were driven out so that they could not return to the community with the plague or other evil that had been transferred to them.

Occasionally the difference was in the style of life pursued by the chosen victim. Frazer again remarks on the ritual practised in Siam where a 'debauched' woman was carried on a litter through the city. During the journey she was pelted with missiles and insults were hurled at her. Outside the city walls she was

thrown onto a dunghill and forbidden to return. The city's badness had been symbolically cast onto the refuse heap.

The motif of difference in the choice of scapegoats was maintained by the Greeks. The Athenians kept a stock of potential
scapegoats, all of whom were characterised by being ugly or
deformed in some way. These degraded and so-called 'useless'
individuals were maintained at public expense, fed and cared for,
but when catastrophe threatened they were haled forth to propitiate the gods. First they were beaten on the genitals with
branches of wild fig, then driven through the city streets and
stoned to death or near death and then burnt. The citizens, who
would all have taken part in this ritual, could then return to their
homes conscious that they had done all in their power to avert
the evil influence.

The Greeks did not always refer to their stocks of the 'different'
when a scapegoat was required, as the scapegoat was occasionally
a volunteer who was bedecked, symbolically loaded with the sins
or fears of the people of the city, led around the streets for all
to see and eventually stoned to death outside the boundary walls.

It is assumed that such volunteers believed that their behaviour
earned them credit not just in the eyes of their fellow citizens
but also in the estimation of their gods. They believed that by
dying in such a way they were gaining merit and doing public
good.

The Romans pursued a similar ritual in which a selected man
was clad in skins, processed through the city streets, beaten with
long white rods by the dancing priests, the Salii, and driven out.

The elimination of disease

The *Standard Dictionary of Folklore, Mythology and Legend*
offers evidence that the practice of ridding communities of disease
by means of a scapegoat was widespread. Until recent times the
Quechua and Aymara Indians used methods for this purpose
which can be traced back to the Incas. When a village was suffering from an epidemic, a black llama was loaded with the clothing
of the sick and driven from the village, carrying the disease with
it. The dictionary also notes that the medicine men of the Quechua and Aymara usually, though not always, transferred the
diseases of their patients to a guinea pig. The unfortunate animal
was then killed and burnt.

An interesting element of this practice is the indifference to the fate of those who consumed the contaminated food or touched the clothing left by the riverside, for it was assumed that they would bear away the disease or evil which permeated the food and clothing. Later we shall see that this process of contamination became part of a contract with people known as sin-eaters who, for a consideration, deliberately took food and clothing supposedly containing the evil, disease, badness or whatever of the recently dead before burial. The indiscriminate disposal of disease became, in the case of the sin-eater, a business.

> During the Crusades, for example, or during its wars with Protestantism, the Catholic Church emphasised the tribal aspects of its doctrine, defining itself primarily by means of its declared adversary, by *projecting* the 'infidel' or the 'heretic' as scapegoat.
>
> (Baigent *et al.* 1986: 160)

There is no doubt that many times throughout history problems that are directly the result of bad government, political miscalculation or even catastrophe and national disaster have been successfully blamed by those who were responsible for dealing with such matters onto specially selected groups of people. The Jews have fallen into this category many times and have suffered the consequences.

Even at this size of operation the scapegoats have many of the characteristics of individuals occupying the same role in smaller groupings. For instance, the communities chosen are generally seen as weak and unable to retaliate. But, more importantly perhaps, the larger community of which the scapegoats are a distinct part bears them great hostility, usually based upon a perception of difference and upon ignorance and dislike. Myths spring up not around similarities but around differences and often serve to emphasise those particular characteristics that are common to a particular race, tribe or people. By contrast, such emphasis on a commonality automatically highlights the differences of the in-group from others, who, if they should be part of the larger community, may be tolerated but their differences are always visible, always available to be used to provide a comparison of deficiency and thus become mythologised by the host community.

Such myths derive their impetus and energy from insecurity, from blindness, from prejudice – and from the wilful creation of a scapegoat.

(Baigent *et al.* 1986: 160)

The true basis of the scapegoating process is here, only writ very large. A society finds that something is going wrong and when they are unwilling to attempt to discover the real causes of their problems, just as in a small group, the search for someone or something to blame usually finds what it seeks in available people who may be already disliked but who are inevitably seen as different. In essence what is created is a survival myth which more or less successfully attributes the problems and failures of an entire people not to any reality of its own social behaviour, structure or organisation but to those elements within itself which are or can be regarded as alien or deficient. The myth may originally have had some basis in fact, but in its fully developed state it can often be seen as a kind of deflection, a distraction from the reality and from any consideration of the actual causes of distress. Its main purpose may be – as in the small group – to maintain the group in existence, but, as nearly every case of this form of scapegoating shows, the relief from distress obtained by scapegoating a relatively if not totally innocent entity is almost always transient, and the problem recurs after a period of time.

In traditional societies manifestations of non-human power and non-biological movements in nature tend to be associated with supernatural powers.

(Cuppitt 1985: 37)

A common form of the transfer of blame is to be found in the treatment that was meted out to so-called witches. The *Malleus Maleficarum* appeared in 1486 and gave details of the behaviour of witches, the signs by which they could be detected, the methods of interrogation and of punishment. In strongly religious societies in western Europe in the fifteenth century, a belief in evil was an absolute article of faith as the counterbalance to a belief in good, the Devil and his minions – the opposite of God and his angels. The belief system was so strong an influence, and the possibility of rational explanation so remote, that it is not surprising that it took the particular form it did and that witch hunting became a frenzied hysteria.

> As the increased spiritual awareness of the Reformation brought a corresponding sensitivity to the ever-present powers of Satan, the mania increased and any misfortune – a tree struck by lightning, a calf born dead – set off a search for a witch. Neighbour distrusted neighbour, and no one was safe from suspicion.
>
> (Edith Simon 1967: 164)

In ordinary people the fear of evil, once again regarded as tangible and transferable, was so powerful and the understanding of the natural causes of events so entirely absent, that the causes for all apparently inexplicable events were automatically attributed to magic. That the causes were inexplicable was almost entirely due to ignorance. Edith Simon (1967: 163) writes:

> Such misfortunes as a brewer's beer spoiling, a farmer's crops failing, babies crying continually or wives falling in love with the wrong husbands were clear evidence that witches were doing the Devil's work.

This ignorance produced an argument which appointed evil, either incarnate or not, as the central cause of misfortune. Its direction towards specific individuals and situations was therefore attributed to the agents of evil who would be either demons or other non-corporeal entities or human beings whose allegiance to the Devil was similar in all respects to that of worthy people to God, except that it was conceived of as being wholly reversed. There were therefore witches and warlocks who had the ability to visit evil upon whomsoever they chose, or as directed by their master.

Another aspect of this belief in evil was that a different kind of beneficial magic was available which brought the fulfilment of wishes, cures and, of course, the promotion of luck. Many people were not averse to the use of the evil power of witches and were prepared to pay for curses to be placed upon the heads of their enemies.

The essential fact of this process for our purposes is that witches, and other dealers in supernatural powers, were prime targets of blame in any village community when things went wrong, whether this was an individual event or occurrences of much wider significance. There is little doubt that many innocent people were killed because they had operated as fortune tellers or suppliers of charms and potions. The communities in which they lived had invested them with magical powers because they needed to believe that some help was available when required, but such people were immediately the focus of blame if anything went wrong.

Witches had many of the attributes of the potential scapegoat. They were often isolated, feared for their supposed powers and, as a result, quite often heartily disliked. Their powers of retaliation, although feared, were seen as limited and as they were usually elderly women, physically non-existent. Thus, if the crops failed the witch was to blame; if animals became sick, the witch was to blame.

Of course this is a simplification but it stresses a factor that is consistent in many forms of scapegoating. Where ignorance of the actual causes of distress and harm exists, then human beings inevitably seek for an explanation. It is as if individuals, groups and communities cannot tolerate or live with events that are apparently inexplicable. Thus, when such events occur no relief, no cleansing can take place until some acceptable explanation has been found. Where witches flourished there was an unshakable belief in supernatural agencies, hence the inexplicable found an explanation in their operation. Since most things that were regarded as inexplicable were also harmful and deleterious, the supernatural agencies were considered to be evil.

The persecution of witches (some historians estimate that during the witch-hunting craze in Germany alone some 100,000 people were killed as witches) is one of the clearest examples of selected members of a society – who were barely tolerated for some of the good things they could do – becoming innocent victims and being blamed for natural events, the causes of which the population as a whole did not and could not understand. It is a prime example of the irrational/transfer form of scapegoating.

Of course, the ideas of magic and of supernatural powers have not entirely died out with the increasing knowledge that science has put at the disposal of everyone.

Today interest in the so-called occult is more widespread than ever before. Popular sun-sign astrology is a subject for light conversation, self-appointed 'Perfect Masters' have attracted large followings, and in almost every large city of Europe and North America there are groups of cultists who claim they are practising authentic witchcraft.

(King 1975: 7)

There may be many who find it easy to accept that events and things they do not understand can be controlled by the powers of magic. Unfortunately it is much easier to blame such powers for consequences that are either harmful or benign than to discover the actual causes. Fear plays as large a part in this process as it has through all the forms of scapegoating that we have recorded.

It is interesting to note that Tyndale, living not many years after the production of the *Maleficarum*, would have been very familar with the concepts of the transfer of blame, of witchcraft and of magic, but whether he believed in such things is another matter.

Sin-eaters

Another professional who might turn up at a funeral in Wales and the border counties was the Sin-eater. According to John Aubrey (who said that the custom was in decline in the 17th century), this character would be outside the house of the deceased as the coffin was carried out and, on receiving a loaf of bread, a maple bowl of beer and sixpence, agreed to take on himself all the sins of the dead person.

(Pegg 1981: 124)

At the opposite end of the size continuum from the victimisation of a whole people there have always been individuals who were willing to operate as scapegoats and, indeed, made a business of it in particular situations. The sin-eater was a common enough phenomenon up to the late 1600s and persisted even longer in parts of Wales and in the Scottish Islands. The ceremony or ritual was simple enough, but contained the essential element of the transfer of evil. The sin-eater, classified by Pegg as a 'professional', was not only a volunteer but one who was paid for his services.

The essentials of the ritual, as described by Aubrey and others, was that food, usually in the form of a loaf of bread, was either passed over the corpse or laid upon its chest. During this contact or proximity the sins of the dead person were believed to inhere in the bread, which was then consumed by the sin-eater. The gossip's bowl full of beer and the sixpence constituted the fee usually received. Believing as they did that the dead would need to go through a long period of purgatory and may even return to walk the earth if their sins were great, this was considered a small enough price to pay for freedom from fear and for relieving the dead of part of their burden.

How the sin-eater discharged his acquired sins no one has yet recorded. One can only assume that the individuals who performed such a service had some sense that the risk they took was one that they had discovered pragmatically to be of a supportable nature. If sin-eaters had in fact been visited with enormous punishment for their pains, I doubt the practice would have lasted as long as it did or been so universal in one form or another. It is not the deterioration of the belief of the transferability of sins that has markedly diminished over time, but the perceived necessity for doing so.

Whipping boys

The phenomenon of the whipping boy marks a notable change in the process of scapegoating. It brings into play a deliberate and conscious substitution in which an entirely innocent person receives punishment on behalf of the person who earned it. But another important factor that establishes the basis for a great deal of public scapegoating today is the concept of the 'relative value' or 'worth' of different individuals.

As we noted in Chapter 1, a whipping boy was an individual who was kept to be whipped when a young prince's behaviour deserved chastisement. The person of the prince was sacrosanct but even princes had to be schooled and to learn that certain behaviours merited punishment, so that punishment was meted out to the substitute – the whipping boy. History offers some named examples of this process in operation.

Barnaby Fitzpatrick served as whipping boy to Edward VI and Mungo Murray performed the same function for Charles I. In 1593, Henry IV of France abjured his Protestant faith and became a Catholic. D'Ossat and Du Perron, who were Henry's ambassadors at the time of his reception into the Roman Catholic Church, were dispatched to Rome to receive whatever punishment the pope decided Henry should suffer. They were ordered to kneel in the portico of St Peter's and sing the miserere. At each verse they were beaten about the shoulders with a switch. Both whipping boys eventually became cardinals.

From the status of princes and their right not to be punished for wrong-doing is derived the idea that certain individuals are of such value to the community, organisation or group that it is inappropriate to diminish, tarnish or in any way impair their value by subjecting them to punishment for wrong-doing. Others, deemed to be of lesser value, are thus selected to receive punishment in their stead. If the evaluation of worth is indeed correct, then some justification may be adduced for this behaviour, but there are many instances where the assessment of value has been purely selfish and personal and the process of substitution an exercise of the use of power to prevent exposure. The process then becomes morally indefensible.

THE GROWTH OF SUPERSTITION

Religious change is forced because, whether we like it or not, religious meanings are changed by changes in the surrounding culture; and the tendency of such forced, involuntary change has generally been to degrade faith into superstition.

(Cuppitt 1985: 11)

During the fifteenth century in particular, superstition grew at a fantastic rate. It was a period when, as Simon (1967: 11) writes, 'there were few dependable scientific laws; the arbitrary miracles of divine omnipotence obtained instead'. This period, according to Simon, included the Hundred Years War between England and France, peasant revolts, the Black Death and various plagues. Trade diminished, hunger was widespread and the intellectual advance of the Middle Ages was ignored. The agricultural populations ' ... subject to the caprices of nature, have ever been superstitious, prone to propitiate an unfathomable deity with charms and to exorcise malicious demons with curses' (Simon 1967: 11).

Superstition is defined as an irrational belief which is founded on fear and ignorance and is usually expressed in terms of excessive reverence for omens and charms. Although such a belief system was at its most powerful during the fifteenth century, it is still with us in many forms.

The deterioration of religious belief into superstition did not mean that the power of supernatural beings to punish diminished but rather that it diffused to every minor aspect of people's lives. Just as witches became the focus of scapegoating for harmful events, the causes of which were not understood, so the development and continuance of superstition has always offered an inviting prospect of being able to devolve blame onto inhuman factors such as fate or luck or the malice of others.

So superstition can be regarded as a fruitful basis for the scapegoating process, and although major belief systems have moved far towards rational explanations of events, the basis of ignorance, which feeds superstition, is still with us. This may well be partly the fault of the explosion of information and knowledge that has taken place this century, which has almost ensured that although rational explanations of a kind are available about most things they have become so specialised that a lifetime's study is barely enough to ensure even a good grasp of a very small area of interest. This leaves the average person with rather large deficits in understanding or, at best, a very superficial knowledge covering a wide area. The lacunae are therefore filled with a different kind of understanding in which superstition, opinion and tradition play quite considerable parts.

As the basis of superstition is the belief that things occur through the interference of unknown elements, then the basic drive to blame in an irrational way is well founded. Elsewhere I have discussed the near impossibility of humans being able to tolerate the apparently inexplicable, which, coupled with the basic and powerful urge to self-preservation, and thus the necessity to avoid responsibility and blame, creates a strong possibility that any such blame will be redirected onto others.

Children and superstition

The persistence of the belief that evil or badness has a transferable presence is quite well shown in the beliefs of children, found in some relatively surprising areas of behaviour. Iona and Peter Opie in their book *The Language and Lore of Schoolchildren* (1959) give a comparison of the treatment of warts. The first example was taken from *The Natural History of Pliny* and the second, 1990 years later, from a Radnorshire schoolboy in 1953. Pliny's method was ' ... on the first day of the moon, each wart must be touched with a single chick pea, after which, the party must tie up the pease in a linen cloth, and throw it behind him, by adopting this plan, it is thought, the warts will be made to disappear.'

The schoolboy's version employed wheat, which was rubbed onto the wart then wrapped in a parcel big enough for someone to see. It was then left secretly at a cross roads. Clearly in this version, and by implication in Pliny's, the parcels were meant to be discovered by some curious person, picked up, and the warts transferred to the finder.

Many cures in folklore are based upon the idea that if the disease or problem can be transferred to another body or substance, then the subject will be cured if that body or substance is discarded. However simple we may think such beliefs may be, there is no mistaking the fundamental acceptance of contagious magic and the transferability of evil and badness that exists and even flourishes at the present day.

Scapegoating in an industrial society

In the play 'Gaslight' by Patrick Hamilton, written in 1931, the husband tries to convince his wife that she is mad. The play was a portrayal of a form of social behaviour which involved getting a member of a family falsely committed to a mental hospital for the purpose of being able to blame the family misfortunes on that member. Of course, motives were never actually that simple.

Commitment to an institution on petition under the 1890 Lunacy Act carried with it vesting of the control of the 'patient's' property in the committing person or his or her representative. But Brown and Pedder (1979) noted that, in 1763, a committee of the House of Commons had reported that 'some people had been committed to asylums as a way of solving family and social problems'.

This illustrates one of the major developments in the process of scapegoating which had become increasingly evident in the eighteenth and nineteenth centuries and probably constitutes by far the greater part of public scapegoating today – the process becomes a rational survival strategy. It is then based not upon any suggestion of propitiation but almost wholly upon the process of substitution, which was an essential part of some forms of the ancient ritual. The mainspring is a fairly selfish but rational desire to scapegoat others, often palpably innocent of any offence either against an individual or a group, to ensure the continuing safety and position of the scapegoater. The process involves being able to convince significant others that blame is attached to the selected victim and not to the scapegoater, a process that was often initiated and expedited by the simple act of condemning the hapless victim and then speedily removing that person from any possibility of being defended. Commitment to an asylum served this purpose remarkably well in that not only was the victim physically removed, but the process cast grave doubts upon any defence the victim was able to muster on the grounds that he or she had been established as insane by virtue of being in an asylum.

STRATEGIC SCAPEGOATING

With the increase in the strategic use of the scapegoating process as a survival procedure comes the development of what might be called the 'fear of exposure'. The ancients laboured under the belief that they *were* always exposed to the gaze of their gods. Thus they had no fear of the possibility of exposure, only a dread of the consequences, and so they developed techniques to abate these consequences if at all possible. The driving force behind a great deal of public scapegoating in modern times seems to be related to the possibility of exposure, a fear of being found out, a fear that the public image so assiduously created and probably not firmly related to the actual person, will be destroyed. Hence the powerful need to dissemble, to deny with as much authority as possible, to deflect and so look for others to take the blame. In effect a simple process of casting others to the wolves.

Given the intrusive nature of modern media coverage of public persons, this deception is not irrational. The media is, after all, the instrument that is selected to generate public images in the first place, and we have seen the steady development of public personages who are regarded as having so-called presentational skills – in essence an ability to manipulate the media by a carefully chosen image presentation designed to convince the general public that the presented individual possesses attributes which demand their support if not their affection.

The other side of the coin is, of course, that area of investigative and thus intrusive journalism which is currently under such hard scrutiny as a result of its being debased to satisfy the need for audiences in certain areas of the media. However, its main functions have always been: (a) to serve the public interest; (b) to discuss when legitimate image creation, as part of an effort to gain support and backing, has tipped over into deceit, duplicity and fraud and become mainly self-seeking; and (c) to expose the image when it becomes a front for either private or public cheating and a dishonest activity rather than an instrument to ensure the necessary power in order to pursue a legitimate public role.

It cannot have escaped many public figures that the dividing line between image creation and character assassination is very thin and that the concept of investigation in the interest of the public is founded upon a matter of opinion in those with the power to initiate such an investigation.

Hence, the fear of exposure is a powerful incentive to create protection by the use of scapegoating procedures by those likely to be investigated. In simple terms, the process operates by having available someone who can, with reasonable safety, be made the focus of exposure and thus divert it from its true target.

Part II

Social behaviour
Examples and analysis

One of the major differences between the modern (i.e. current) description of the process of scapegoating and the old is the apparently vast increase in complexity. Whereas the ancients appeared to have considered the propitiating and sacrifical aspects of the process to be of paramount importance and the aspect of the victim little considered, current discussion is concerned with concepts of provocation and with the characteristics of victims and their personalities. Another issue that did not bother our ancestors relates to the idea that scapegoating can be a process that is designed specifically to ensure the safety and preservation of a single individual rather than a group or a community. Thus the level of deliberate victimisation of the innocent is much greater, with a consequent increase in selfishness of motivation and a decrease in morality.

A further difference lies in the attempt to understand, which may well be a consequence of the massive reduction in the common perception of any form of divine supervision. Behaviour of all kinds is to be understood in human terms – in motivation, attitudes, background, personality, perceptions, etc. – and it is the opinion of individuals, both separately and *en masse*, that is important rather than the condescension of divine beings.

However, this change from religious ritual to social behaviour may not be what it seems. It may be purely a change in the nature of the evidence available which may, in turn, be dependent upon the changes in the major concerns of society. Among the ancients, ritual religious behaviour was a communal activity and, for all the reasons given earlier, of supreme importance for the maintenance of what was seen as a relatively fragile order supervised by powerful and punishing deities. The activities of the individuals were not regarded as being of any great interest until and unless one of those individuals became uncommon in some manner that impinged upon the structure of the society. Thus the extant records of social behaviour tend to be of major social occasions and of the important people who were involved.

However, the changes in society that are documented begin to bring into focus the behaviour of lower mortals, and the changes in the perceptions of the supervising and regulating powers of divine beings tend to turn the centre of responsibility for behaviour to the institutions of society and, eventually, to small social groups and the individual himself.

Thus, the increasing secularisation of society and the intensification of rational enquiry into all aspects of human existence may well be the prime cause of the deterioration of the ritual nature of the process of scapegoating. With changed concepts of divine beings, the process of scapegoating becomes much more individualistic and is regarded as part of ordinary social behaviour. No longer a ritual to serve the good of the community but much more oriented to the safety and maintenance of the individual, the small group or the organisation. Now the process of victimisation is investigated not just as part of a ritual process but from the point of view of the victim, and thus there grows the beginnings of the idea that some victims are self-selecting.

The chapters in Part II trace these changes and attempt to describe modern processes of scapegoating and being scapegoated, and we look at the various efforts to provide a rational explanation and understanding of what actually happens.

Chapter 4

Scapegoating as public behaviour
The process of scapegoating

When cornered, French politicians are notorious for blaming their neighbours. Just as last year's debate on the Maastricht referendum was dominated by fear of Germany, so Britain appears to be the latest scapegoat for France's economic trials.
(Editorial, the *Daily Telegraph* 1993: 12)

When one state blames another for its economic difficulties and the editors of reputable newspapers can describe the process as scapegoating, then it must be immediately obvious that although some things may be the same about the classical process as named by Tyndale, some other elements have changed almost out of all recognition. At the risk of being blatantly obvious, the main elements that have changed are the societies in which scapegoating is practised and also what might be called 'the element of conscious strategy' that has developed. What has remained essentially the same, and the main reason why it is possible to regard all forms of scapegoating as belonging to the same category of behaviour, is the ubiquitous and everlasting need of human beings to avoid censure and blame.

It is not beyond the bounds of logical possibility that the government of one large European country can accuse another of being the main cause of its economic difficulties. But it is just as possible, in fact more probable, that the first government, or some empowered representative of that government, is making an attempt to shift the blame for what is largely a crisis of their own making onto the second government. The mechanism of such an operation is basically the same as that used by the Jews and described in Leviticus. Hence the editor's use of the word scapegoat to describe what was happening is perfectly legitimate, but how much more difficult is it to be certain of how much actual truth resides in the accusation and how much of it is a rational strategy of displacement and evasion? How much depends upon presenting a rational explanation of what is being done and how much is a device designed solely for the preservation in post of those involved?

CHANGES IN SOCIETY

In this chapter we shall look at some of these difficulties and also at some of the major changes that have occurred in societies: in size; in diversity of peoples, cultures and beliefs; in the enormous increase in secularisation; in the development of rational and non-religious explanations; and in the effect of having constant access to news and information.

Size

> As group size increases, contending forces are unleashed, some foster others hinder group performance.
>
> (Davis 1969: 72)

One indisputable change in communities from those which existed in biblical times is their size.

The small communities of ancient and classical times were very rarely urban and even if they were they tended to be small enough, like the Greek city states, to involve almost the whole population in state occasions. These would include decision-making meetings when war threatened and, certainly, religious ceremonies. Even where one government ruled a large empire, the individual units of which the empire was composed were towns and villages and occasional cities. Most people lived on the land and were, to a large extent, self-supporting. Clans, families and kinship groups formed the basic units of such societies and were the main instruments for passing on traditions, skills and property and in defending the rights of their members.

Modern societies are huge and the bonds of individuals to those societies are probably weak, but without doubt there still exist clans and families and other forms of relational linkages that bind people into fairly close-knit groups. There are also many other forms of relational association for all manner of different purposes concerned with work, education, leisure, belief, etc. The major effect of such an increase in the size of a society has been a diminution of the individual's sense of belonging to it. Indeed, the individual is more likely to feel that he or she is an integral part of some subunit of that society than of the society as a whole. The immediate face-to-face nature of a small social unit – or at least an awareness of the close presence of others, which was such a powerful feature of small total societies – is now to be found most effectively functioning in these smaller subsections of the total society or state. They may be powerful in influencing that total society, or, equally, they may be in confrontation and conflict with it.

As we shall see, the immediate communication that was possible in the small society has been replaced in the large states by other forms of contact which, while they may be as immediate, are no longer a direct personal experience shared with other people. Modern communication systems are selective in content and presentation. The information they contain has been assessed and filtered before it arrives before the consumer. They are also responsible for presenting information about areas that are remote to the people who receive such material. Thus it is not difficult to find members of one society who know something about the affairs of a society thousands of miles away – and perhaps they know even more of that society than they do of their local community.

A considerable amount of public scapegoating is dependent for its form and consequences upon the size of modern communities and equally upon the speed and selectivity of communication systems. Strangely enough, size also emphasises the power of smaller units, probably because they possess greater reality and immediacy for the individual than the larger unit states in which they exist.

Diversity

A second indisputable change from earlier societies has been the increasing diversity of peoples, cultures and beliefs that can be found inside any one state unit. Of course some societies have always been mixed since the beginnings of urbanisation. Rome, in the heyday of the Empire, was extremely cosmopolitan and harboured people from all over Europe and Africa, but such diversity created problems. Few, if any, of these early multi-ethnic communities were democratic organisations and the problems generated by ethnic minorities or peoples with different religions could be treated with either summary brutality or easy tolerance. The different peoples tended to accept the standards of the host nation and it was only when they refused to do so that ruthless suppression occurred. A good example was the cruel treatment the normally tolerant Romans handed out to Christians who refused to acknowledge the Roman gods.

Modern democratic societies which, on the surface, are tolerant and not easily pushed into ruthless suppression, nevertheless do have minority communities where different attitudes, opinions, beliefs, cultures, etc., come in conflict with aspects of the host nation and trouble foments and occasionally erupts. When this happens the pattern of blame shows very clearly most of the signs of the process of scapegoating.

In September 1985 at Handsworth, an area containing several ethnic groups, riots broke out and street battles ensued. Later when the situation was reasonably quiet and the different groups involved began to assess the damage and to allocate blame, the following factors emerged:

- The West Indian community blamed the police for being insensitive. They alleged that they had been harassed by officers and had responded to defend themselves. They also blamed the unrest on the fact that a grossly disproportionate number of their community were unemployed.
- The Indian community blamed the West Indians who, they claimed, were jealous and envious of their standard of living, of their personal wealth which, the Indians claimed, was the result of their own hard work.
- The police blamed greed, criminality and hooliganism, because, as they alleged, these were the behavioural manifestations with which they were faced when the trouble broke.
- The local politicians blamed the government cuts which they said had compelled them to curb expenditure. They also blamed the methods of policing. National politicians of the Left blamed the government's policies, which they said had brought about cuts in provision, unemployment and lack of care. Those of the Right blamed the thuggery of minorities in the area, the nature of ethnic communities (by implication that

they were a natural source of conflict) and greed, because there had been a considerable amount of looting.

- Other elements quoted by various sources suggested that copying the behaviour observed in films and TV programmes was also a responsible element. This went under the general title of 'copycat' behaviour. The presence of reporters and TV cameras at the scene of the riots, the influence of the media and, finally, that the young people of the area did not have enough excitement in their lives and suffered from boredom, were all offered as explanations.

This complex web of allegations is a clear illustration of some of the major problems attendant upon any attempt at analysis of possible scapegoating behaviour. In the widest sense in this scenario all these claims could be true, or at least partially so. Acceptance of any one over the others without real evidence would tend to indicate prejudice and bias.

The first problem then rests upon the extreme difficulty of establishing whether any of the blame-laying accusations rests on a firm basis either of evidence or of belief. Such complex social situations seldom have one clear and powerful motivation, but in order to state that a person, a group or an organisation is being scapegoated it is absolutely essential that there should be clear evidence that the allegations of responsibility and of causation are untrue, or at least partially so. This, in effect, means that any rational and real involvement in causing difficulties and problems is sufficient to dismiss any accusation of scapegoating.

A scapegoat has to be innocent of causing the events, behaviour or situations for which he or she is being blamed.

What is manifestly important, apart from the complexity of a situation like the Handsworth riots, is the fact that it is essential to include evidence not just of provocation or other reason for the behaviour, but also, and most necessary, of belief. Prejudice, opinion, traditional attitudes always exercise enormous influence in shaping the response patterns to perceived threat or frustration. They likewise influence the choice of those who will be blamed, especially when the actual causes are either hidden or unknown or unrecognised for what they are. Many people have been blamed for economic disaster and killed, when in fact the basic reason for being chosen by their killers was that they were different, disliked and their persecutors could find no logical reason for their diminished state that they were able to accept.

This factor is well illustrated in multi-racial societies by the discriminatory choice of victims, apparently based solely on the prejudice and ignorance surrounding racial difference.

Secularisation

It may be appropriate at this point to make a brief comment on the increasing secularisation of western society. The major effect of this process as far as scapegoating is concerned has been to remove the prime cause of problems and difficulties and of punishment and reward which were the province of the deities, and to substitute other factors. Though extremely strong religious beliefs continue to offer the same oversight by divine beings which allowed early societies to develop the rites of propitiation and atonement, the major oversight agencies in modern societies seem to have become the society itself, or some immediately contiguous part of it, and the individual's own conscience and self-image.

The oft-repeated phrase by the character Waldo in Dylan Thomas's *Under Milk Wood*, 'What'll the neighbours say?', clearly illustrates that the scrutiny that most of us bear in mind as we live our lives is seldom that of gods but of those immediately close to us and, in particular, those who have power over our lives or whose opinions are of great worth in our estimation.

As we shall see later, this matter of worth is of great importance as one of the prime undivulged reasons for public scapegoating is concerned with the relative values of the chosen victim and of the public figure his or her sacrifice is designed to protect.

Explanation

Alongside the replacement of the divine supervisor by the secular society and the individual's self-image has been the growth in rational and scientific explanations of natural events. Although, in times of crisis, individuals have a tendency to believe in the intervention of divine beings into their affairs, they no longer seek to protect themselves from disease, epidemics by sacrifice to gods, nor to expiate their wrong-doing by offerings.

That this statement is not wholly true must be immediately

obvious. For what is absolutely commonplace, particularly in western Europe and among those who would not call themselves believers in divine agencies, is a tendency to hedge their bets. They are aware that floods are caused by excess rainfall and geological factors that are perfectly explicable in terms of scientific data, but the acceptance of these rational data is also often accompanied by an irrational belief that the individual has been singled out to be the recipient of this particular catastrophe. Non-believers still ask for the protection of God although, if asked, they would undoubtedly say that they were rationally aware that their protection lay in their own ability to provide for it. Of course, they could also say that chance entered into the calculation. Chance in this instance tends to be equated with luck, but inevitably means the occurrence of events and conditions that are totally unforeseen.

Information

The last of the great changes in societies which we shall consider as having some effect on the form that scapegoating takes, is the immense increase in the availability of information. The place where the influence of information shows most markedly is in the arena of public scapegoating. Consider the following extracts, from some English newspapers, on public scapegoating.

- Child murders: 'Too often the social worker is scapegoated in cases such as child murder, which outrage public opinion' (6 June 1991).
- A football manager: 'From lowly fullback to ultimate fall guy' (24 November 1993).
- International economic affairs: ' ... so Britain appears to be the latest scapegoat for France's economic travails' (6 February 1993).
- An attempt to rehabilitate Philistines: 'A scapegoat untethered' (1 October 1992).
- Locking up suspects: ' ... I hate scapegoating – the school of thought which believes it more important to lock up a suspect than to catch the right one' (Brenda Maddox 1993).
- Wrongly convicted persons: 'scapegoats of Justice' (Christopher Price 1991).
- Politicians: 'Thatcher is just seeking scapegoats, says Lawson' (1993).

What is revealed about public scapegoating in these brief captions is as follows:

- Certain people are exposed to an increased possibility of being blamed by virtue of the role they occupy.
- The likelihood of scapegoating increases enormously when the exposed persons are dealing with areas of public life in which, when disaster strikes, public outrage and great frustration is generated.
- Exposure of public persons is made a great deal more likely by the activities of investigative media people.
- There is a recognition by the general public that a considerable amount of public scapegoating is a self-preservation gambit.

The case of Beverly Allitt, a 25-year-old nurse, illustrates most of the points about public scapegoating and also interestingly enough the failure of the process to transfer blame.

In February and April 1991 Beverly Allitt killed four children and injured nine others. She worked as a nurse on the children's ward of the Grantham and Kesteven hospital for only two months. At her trial in 1993 she received 13 life sentences.

Sir Henry Clothier, who conducted a private enquiry into the situation, said of Allitt that she was 'the malevolent cause of the unexpected collapses of children'. Although others criticised the overworked doctors, the shortage of nurses and a weak hospital management, the report emphasised that proper staffing levels would not have prevented Allitt's actions but it might have made them more difficult to achieve. The report had been expected to scapegoat staff at the hospital. Many people could not see how such events could have taken place unnoticed.

Sir Henry Clothier was reported in the national press of 12 February 1994 as saying:

> But those who read the report will see that many months ago we warned ourselves against the danger of laying blame merely to assuage the grief and anger of innocent people at the wrongs done to them by Beverly Allitt. When we have found fault we have plainly said so without fear or favour.

The parents of some of the children wanted to know why the managers had not been disciplined. They complained that the two consultant paediatricians in charge of the ward when Allitt worked there, and two nursing managers, had been made scapegoats while the senior management criticised in the report were still employed in the Health Service. The medical staff referred to by the parents were Dr Charith Nanayakkara and Dr Nelson Porter, both of whom had been made redundant in 1993 ostensibly because of the transfer of the management of paediatric services to the Queen's Medical Centre at Nottingham; Sister Barbara Barker was made redundant and the clinical services manager Mrs Moira Onions took early retirement.

Under the heading NO NEED FOR SCAPEGOATS sections of the press stated that the report did not make the assumption that the tragedy was avoidable and did not place the moral and legal responsibility on those who failed to prevent it.

The primary explanation of the events was given as Allitt's wickedness, but there was still a bitter campaign of recrimination. Most of those involved thought that the consultant paediatricians should not be condemned as if they shared the guilt of murder.

It was also generally held that they had been sacrificed by the Health Authority, despite the fact that the report was an attempt to apportion 'real' blame and thus to reduce the development of scapegoating. By the time the report was published, however, it was already too late to reverse any decisions.

This tragic affair highlighted some important points. The Allitt case was clear; cause-and-effect responsibility and blame are all too horribly obvious. What is most important is how blame was apportioned between those who were generally regarded as having failed to prevent such a monstrous series of events occurring. Whether or not the Health Authority action in making the two consultants and two other staff redundant was designed to imply that these people were responsible is not relevant. What is relevant is that the public and, to some extent, the media thought they were being offered as sacrifices to enable the matter to be closed at the cost of four people's careers and, in some cases, their present and future quality of life.

There may have been some culpability on the part of the four who had been dispensed with, but the public, and in particular the parents of the children from the ward in the Grantham and Kesteven hospital, believed that others infinitely more responsible in their eyes were still in employment. It is a remarkable fact about public scapegoating that when the public believe they are being offered scapegoats, deflective shields, they tend to reject those offered and search for those they would define as the 'real' culprits.

One of the problems in this case which exacerbated that rejection was that the Clothier enquiry was held in secret. No matter how accurately the report's conclusions delineate what occurred and the factors of negligence, bad management or whatever, there is little chance that they, or the sacrifice of the four staff, will be accepted. The death of children is always a highly charged and emotional affair. When they die by being murdered in the supposedly intensely caring environment of a children's ward in a hospital, then the emotion is powerful indeed. No amount of cold fact will obliterate the overwhelming need to blame. Allitt was found guilty, so she cannot be much of a focus for blame because she is obviously grossly disturbed. Thus the blame must go to those who should have prevented her from being able to take such lethal actions.

The fact that some have apparently been sacrificed to shield others who are generally held to be much more responsible, and that most people realise this, indicates that this particular deflective exercise of scapegoating has failed in its basic purpose.

> However, at times of crisis, there is a public clamour for more tangible scapegoats from the ranks of the elite that is held responsible for some misfortune.
>
> (Kraupl-Taylor 1964: 15)

Given that a crisis can indeed put the 'elite', as Kraupl-Taylor calls them, under considerable pressure to admit their responsibility it is perhaps only to be expected that they, the 'elite', will seek others who can be offered in their place to fulfil the desire to see heads roll. It is almost irrelevant whether such selectees have any involvement whatsoever with the crisis. All that really matters is that the victims can be made to appear guilty, carry the blame and, of course, be unable to vindicate themselves. In the Allitt case this latter essential did not hold.

THREAT AND CRISIS

What we have been discussing is the response to threat, particularly in the midst of some form of crisis. Some further study of threat and crisis should prove useful in our attempt to understand scapegoating procedures.

References to threat in the psychological literature are scarce and the concept of survival even more so. Yet how else is it possible to describe the reaction of scapegoaters except to say that they perceive some threat to their survival which they attempt to deflect by focusing the source of the threat onto another person?

Ordinary people continually perceive threat in their everyday existence, often in the form of possible painful consequences. Change and the unfamiliar – particularly when these are introduced arbitrarily and unexpectedly and without prior consultation – have been proved to assume life-threatening dimensions and to provoke resentment, fear, anger and, above all, resistance.

Most of the examples of scapegoating offered here demonstrate a clear response to fear or to some form of threat. This is particularly so as we have seen of individuals in public life who have a considerable amount to lose by being exposed in some way or other in detrimental fashion. Such exposure has all the characteristics of change, and particularly unwelcome change at that. It is inspired and initiated from without; it is about to generate a perceived loss for the individual at its focus; it is unsought and has every possibility of destroying cherished ambitions.

Straightforward denial and defiance appears to have little chance of being successful and it is almost inevitable that deflection techniques will be brought into play. The principal one, of course, is to set up another to take the blame, thus creating a scapegoat; another is to find a crisis of superior dimensions and interest. Regarding this last factor, Raven and Rubin (1976: 124) remind us that the impact of a common threat can be so powerful that it overrides even very strong negative feelings and prejudices.

In essence, this kind of scapegoating – which we can call 'deflective' and rational – tends to be the outcome of a crisis situation and the stages of crisis development can show clearly how such a point of action is reached.

> The essential factor influencing the occurrence of a crisis is an imbalance between the difficulty and importance of the problem and the resources immediately available to deal with it.
>
> (Caplan 1964: 39)

Stage 1.   A situation arises which generates tension and

	brings into play the habitual and usual problem-solving responses.
Stage 2.	The usual response patterns fail to deal with the situation and the tension increases.
Stage 3.	The rise in tension generates the energy needed to go beyond the usual response formula and can be used:

(a) to redefine the problem;
(b) to discover new ways of coping with it;
(c) to redefine the priorities of certain goals in the light of the continued existence of the problem.

This may result in the problem being solved or at least mitigated.

If the problem is not solved, the level of frustration will tend to push the individual to a level of disorganisation that can result in attempts to use relief methods which would previously have been wholly unacceptable, e.g. the deflection of blame and responsibility onto some other innocent person.

It is feasible that this process can also function when the focal point is not an individual but a group. The fear of punishment must be one of humanity's primary fears.

> Without fear of punishment, the majority of people would behave less socially than they actually do, for the super-ego does not entirely replace real persons in authority.
>
> (Alexander 1948: 144)

However, it must also be agreed that other fears – of appearing foolish, or ignorant or inept; of failure; of loss of self-esteem, or status or position – all follow close behind. The fear of losing something that we value or hold to be worth while is also very important.

Even if the loss actually occurs there is some solace to be had in being able to blame someone and/or something for that loss. It is, however, inevitable that a very strong drive can arise from the need to prevent that loss occurring in the first place. So there is an equally strong desire to seek out those culpable in order to vent anger, resentment and hurt upon them and to evade any self-examination and soul searching that might discover the real causes of loss.

If loss is a factor in laying blame, so is fear. The ancients feared punishment by their all-seeing gods; moderns fear not an all-seeing public but one that can be informed through the power of exposure. Mistakes are made and costs incurred. Inevitably responsibility for costs which are unwanted and damaging is laid at the feet of those who are supposed to have brought them about. As the studies of prejudice have so often shown, those chosen to take this blame are not usually the people who are actually responsible but are simply available, have some basic and essential differences that are very noticeable, and are possibly intensely disliked.

Aronson (1980) believed that prejudice produced a modern form of scapegoating. Indeed, he offered a 'scapegoat theory of prejudice'. His thesis was in essence one of displacement in that the people for whom frustration was inexpressible in relation to its cause, chose to vent that frustration upon groups who were visible, relatively powerless and disliked before the frustration arose. This particular thesis is as much concerned with the manner of choosing victims as with the reasons for the scapegoating process, an issue we shall examine later.

Because the times we live in have become characterised by the need to explain behaviour in rational ways, the process of scapegoating – as might be expected – has attracted considerable attention from social scientists of all kinds. One such professional, F. Kraupl-Taylor, introduced the ideas of the 'purifying scapegoat' and the 'malefactor scapegoat' into his writing.

Of these, the first is immediately recognisable as the traditional scapegoat, a being onto whom evil was transferred thus purifying and cleansing the person or group from whom the evil was removed. But Kraupl-Taylor's second category of malefactor scapegoat is rather different in that it is based upon the belief that evil is not concrete and transferable but is basically a form of intended behaviour. He writes: 'The motif is therefore not concerned with magic manoeuvres of transferring evil, but with evil doers and their punishment.' He is drawing a distinction between evil, which has an existence in its own right irrespective of where it might be temporarily lodged or made manifest, and human behaviour, which is like all other behaviour in that it is purposeful, i.e. intended to achieve relatively specific outcomes. In this particular form of behaviour, these could be described as evil outcomes.

I suppose that to be precise it should be clearly stated that the 'evil' of the outcome is how it would be described by the recipients of the behaviour and probably by any interested and knowledgeable observers. The outcomes for the perpetrator may well be extremely rewarding. According to Kraupl-Taylor (1964: 14) such practitioners are punished

> for two incompatible reasons. Their punishment can be regarded as a safety device that propitiously deflects the same fate from us for the sins we ourselves have committed. Alternatively, their punishment can be viewed as a preventive device that obviates further malefaction by either the original culprit or others.

Certain people are more likely to be exposed by the nature of the matters with which they deal. Politicians of all kinds are an obvious example and illustrations abound of such people being blamed for events that occurred within the area of their responsibility which may or may not have been brought about by their actions. But there are others, e.g. social workers, who deal with human problems at the more disastrous end of the scale of seriousness, such as the murder of a child, which can occasion such a great deal of public interest that the deficiencies of practice suddenly become the focus of intense public outcry.

Margaret Leslie (1991) quoted Professor Colin Pritchard,

> There is this great public need to blame someone and it is polifically expedient not to criticise the police or other professions.

The problem with social workers is that they fulfil too many of the criteria of selection for the scapegoat role. For instance, the public image of social workers is not good; there is little understanding of their social role; they are immediately available for blame because (a) they claim to have the power to deal with crises, (b) they enter people's homes and (c) they make judgements about affairs that very closely affect ordinary people who have their own cherished beliefs about what is right and proper. In particular, they are involved with the most vulnerable people in society. Therefore, when a child is found battered to death and social workers have had a connection with the family, inevitably they are blamed for not preventing such an appalling tragedy. The fact that the child may have been killed by one or other of its parents seems to be such an unacceptable fact that blame attaches less to the actual perpetrators than to those who are deemed to have failed to prevent the occurrence of the event.

The logic of this is remarkable and has to be based upon factors other than the actual incident of a child's murder. There is a strong element about the outrage that contains some understanding that parents can be driven beyond the limits of their control by circumstances and the behaviour of children. A murderer's behaviour, while never forgiven, is something that most parents can understand. It follows, therefore, that it is not the parent who should carry the blame but those who appear to the ordinary person to have been employed to prevent such things happening. The social worker by virtue of his or her role, by virtue of being involved in the crises of human existence, is the culprit chosen by the public for the focus of anger, guilt and blame. This is almost a straight projection of ubiquitous fears each person may have about their potential for similar behaviour.

What the media and others label scapegoating in public life is obviously different in some of its features from the scapegoating that happens in families and in other small groups. For instance, public figures are frequently cast in the role of scapegoat and thus suffer the consequences. There is also a form of public scapegoating which starts with some part of the population accusing some public figure of being responsible for events that have produced damaging effects in their lives, but instead of the public figure suffering the ignominy of this attack, he or she is able to deflect the opprobrium of the damaged public onto some other person, persons or events and, if successful, escape all consequences.

This process of deflection has two important factors. First, if the chosen victim is innocent of any complicity in the events for which the public figure is being attacked, then he or she becomes a genuine scapegoat. However, such is the complexity of the allocation of responsibility within public institutions, this innocence can seldom be proved with any degree of certainty even if an enquiry into the matter is held at a later date. Blame is often then apportioned on the basis of available evidence. As we shall see later, there is also involved the same constituent which existed in the use of whipping boys – that is, the overall worth of the public figure is so great that whether actually responsible or not it is often deemed necessary to sacrifice some comparatively innocent person in order to maintain the public figure in a position in which he or she can continue to function.

Of course, the victim so selected may be another member of the organisation to which the public figure belongs, or may be entirely outside it. Indeed, the scapegoat may not even be a person, but an event or a set of circumstances. For instance, the general public blamed the government for the harshness of the recession, believing this to be entirely due to ministerial mismanagement. The government selected for its scapegoat the stringencies imposed upon it by its membership of the ERM. This was an external scapegoat, and as the Common Market had often been used in this capacity the accusation of blame may well have contained enough truth to make it appear valid.

Sometime later, when the economic situation did not improve – at least in the eyes of the general public – the government sacrificed its chancellor, Norman Lamont. Ostensibly the excuse given was that his relationship with the media was injudicious and damaging. In effect, whatever else may have triggered the decision he was offered as a scapegoat, one who could be blamed quite logically for what had gone wrong.

A great deal of scepticism was expressed about this manoeuvre but without doubt it eased the pressure of complaint as there were also beginning to be signs that the worst of the recession was over.

Sometimes the process involves a kind of chain reaction that is different in kind from the displacement process we shall look at later. Displacement involves the dissipation of tension caused by frustration and operates by discharging that tension onto some other available individual. The chain form of public scapegoating seems to produce not just relief from tension but exoneration from blame at all stages in the chain except the last.

The whole process of public scapegoating can be described as a diversionary process where the sole purpose is to deflect blame past the actual people responsible for problems and have it placed on others. While this may well succeed with public figures, it is often less successful when communities blame others for what are essentially problems of their own making. What happens in this instance is purely an attempt to hide, to obfuscate crises. Depending upon the degree to which the ploy is operated by those who know the real problems, it is devious and expedient and, as we shall see later, a temporary measure. If the time gained by the expedient is used to deal with the actual causes then it may well turn out to have been beneficial. If, on the other hand, it becomes a long-term effort and self-sustaining, then the original causes will tend to remain – apart, that is, from any large unforeseen consequences that may occur.

With regard to the obfuscation process, Bernard-Henri Levy gave an example while writing about the collapse of the ERM when the French blamed the Germans and the Germans blamed the French.

> The truth is that the argument has suddenly lost any real importance. This agitation in politics and the media, this frantic search for someone to blame, for a scapegoat, seems above all to have had the effect of obscuring the real question – which is not about causes but consequences, and the meaning of the crisis that has befallen us.
>
> (The *Daily Telegraph*, August 1993: 14)

Levy is here hinting that the whole process of scapegoating, of blame allocation is not just one of evasion of responsibility but also one of obscuring the essential problem. Of course, hiding under a flurry of blaming and diverting attention is an extremely clever ploy for evading responsibility because, unlike straightforward denial or buck-passing, it appears to be constructive in its apparent search for causes. But like all solutions to problems that are founded in wrongly assessed or just inaccurate assumptions of causation, it merely brings about a situation that not only cannot deal with the real and actual causes but entails other consequences based on the pursuit of false solutions. In the meantime, of course, the scapegoats suffer and the real culprits, both situational and individual, remain unscathed.

If it is generally true that the consequences that are considered when initiating behaviour are mainly those that might be called immediate and apparent, then it is also true that those that occur sometime into the future are seldom considered. Thus when such distant consequences actually occur they often catch the person who initiated the sequence completely off guard. Take the case of Paddy Ashdown, presented in greater detail in Chapter 5. When he became involved with his secretary he was not the leader of his party. He was a politician and a fairly prominent public figure, but intelligent as he is, did he consider the possible effects of his behaviour on his family, his colleagues and his public image should it ever become public knowledge? Five years after the event circumstances that were highly unpredictable at the time exposed behaviour that was previously hidden, largely forgotten and probably considered innocuous. The point is that when this kind of event occurs to those who have a public image to maintain, there has to be a strong tendency to evade the consequences by laying the blame elsewhere, though Mr Ashdown to his credit did not do this.

This, however, introduces another point. Human beings are not very good at predicting consequences. With the best will in the world the information available at any given moment is seldom adequate in kind, quality, order or quantity to make accurate predictions except in limited areas over short periods of time and with some calculation of the probable margin of error. But, of course, it would be wholly incapacitating to adventure nothing on the basis that even if the desired outcome was to be achieved, so many other more important consequences, which could not be foreseen, would also occur.

In this way we have to enter into actuarial calculations where the probability of something actually occurring can be calculated on the basis of an analysis of past experience, current situation and the extrapolation of trends. This kind of exercise may be ideal for business, but it is hardly applicable to everyday social affairs. Planners of all kinds are aware that even this kind of calculation is not remarkably efficient because of the large number of variables that are either incalculable or difficult to assess.

What we are left with at this point are two quite simple facts. First, the long-term consequences of behaviour are extremely difficult if not impossible to calculate and, second, as a result, we are continually being taken by surprise by events which appear to be random but, with hindsight, are not.

The element of surprise, when it occurs, occasions a defensive response frequently manifesting itself in the form of a displacement of responsibility, a scapegoating process or sometimes by an appeal to the logic of explanation or by a profession of ignorance.

One final point about public scapegoating is the effect that it produces on the behaviour of others. The way public figures behave establishes norms of behaviour for the general public, particularly if a great deal of media exposure is given to certain events. In a complex and diverse society there are many available models of apparently acceptable behaviour, but in order to exert influence they have to be known to those who will be influenced. This is one of the main reasons why TV, films and the media generally are often held responsible for establishing patterns of behaviour – especially those that are unacceptable.

Chapter 5

Scapegoating as social behaviour
Examples of the process of scapegoating in families, organisations and groups

Often the roles which get played out in a group are projections of the disowned part of the other members' personality. Scapegoating is an example of this. When any one person in a group carries the role of 'victim', the leader can make a group level intervention to get the members to consider what is being avoided by having someone in the group act out that part of themselves.

(Elaine Kepner 1980: 21)

This chapter offers examples of scapegoating in the family, organisations and groups and attempts to analyse the process, with the intent of showing how the norms of scapegoating behaviour displayed in public life, and available to all, appear in other human gatherings and are accepted and modified, being less public and based in smaller units. However, the basic need to evade blame and consequence still provides the most powerful and fundamental drive.

SCAPEGOATING IN THE FAMILY

This pattern (*scapegoating*) is a special case of a common phenomenon, the achievement of group unity through the scapegoating of a particular member.

(Bell and Vogel 1970: 382)

Bell and Vogel see the process of scapegoating in the family as one of maintenance: that is, as a process which stops the problems within the family splitting it apart. As we shall be looking at this process in some detail in Chapters 7 and 9, it will suffice here simply to describe the process as portrayed by Bell and Vogel.

In the course of their research, these authors noted that in the families in their survey, the member selected to become the family scapegoat was usually a child. In so-called 'well' families used as controls, the tensions that were generated were dealt with in ways that did not involve the use of a family member as a victim. Either the tension in these families was less than the families with scapegoats or they had successfully developed non-pathological methods of coping. When a child did become a scapegoat then that child was often presented as being emotionally disturbed so that the clinical picture was that of a family *with* a disturbed child.

Bell and Vogel were concerned that this simple picture actually concealed the fact that the emotional disturbance presented by the child was due in no small measure to being the focus for the conflicts and tensions of the other family members. Indeed, they began to believe that the reason that such a family was able to tolerate those conflicts and tensions lay solely with the selected child, who was actually absorbing them, who not only became disturbed as a consequence but was also the lynch pin in an equilibrium which allowed the family to continue to function.

Bell and Vogel describe their paper, entitled, 'The emotionally disturbed child as the family scapegoat', by saying it 'is concerned with how a child in the family, the emotionally disturbed child, was used as a scapegoat for the conflicts between parents, and what the functions and dysfunctions of this scapegoating are for the family' (p. 383).

An analysis of this paper produced the following elements of the process of scapegoating in the family.

Tension

General

- Tensions not satisfactorily resolved.
- Deep fears about the marital relationship.
- Deep fears about the partner's behaviour.
- Each felt that they could not predict responses.
- Responses were thought to be of great importance and to be potentially damaging.
- Each felt that they could not communicate directly, and if they could it would be dangerous.
- Each resorted to manipulation and to masking and evasion.

Sources

- The personality problems of the spouses.
- The conflict of cultural value orientations – each had been socialised into different cultural patterns.
- The relationship of the family to the larger community which tended to force them back into themselves.
- The relationship to the family of origin, each showed attachment to own parents and antagonism to spouse's parents.

These sources of conflict and tension could not be contained without some discharge. The families tended to internalise the standards of the communities in which they lived and were thus unable to find any legitimate basis for scapegoating and blaming anyone outside the family; they were therefore obliged to choose a member of the family.

Selection of the scapegoat

The main factors influencing selection were:

- The relative powerlessness of the child *vis-à-vis* the parents.
- The need to choose someone who was not performing any essential family role.
- The need to choose a person intimately related to the sources of tension.
- The choice should be able to symbolise the conflicts by, for example:
(a) a lack of achievement, failure
(b) acting independently and violating the family norms of loyalty
(c) gender – if the problems were about family males then the child chosen was male
(d) age – if the problems concerned older members then an older child was selected
(e) the chosen one usually had some marked resemblance to one or other parent in mannerisms or behaviour.
- The choice usually was of lower intelligence than other members.
- The choice usually had suffered serious physical disease when young or had a striking physical abnormality.

Bell and Vogel also found that where no appropriate choice was available then a large cognitive distortion occurred so that a child who was just physically present within the family could be selected to symbolise the tensions – in other words, to become representative of them – and was then scapegoated. Older children seemed to be the preferred objective in this case.

Induction into scapegoat role

The choice has to carry out the role of 'problem child'.

The parents explicitly criticise but they also support the chosen victim and encourage him or her to perform the allotted role, e.g. by

- failing to carry through threats;
- delaying punishment;
- displaying indifference to and acceptance of the symptoms;
- displaying an unusual interest in the symptoms;
- offering gratification to the child because of the symptoms, e.g special attention, exemption from certain responsibilities;
- offering inconsistency of encouragement between parents.

Once the victim was stabilised in the scapegoat role and disturbed state it meant that the role could not easily be passed to another child or other member of the family.

Consequences

Functionally what occurred was a relatively stable state of family equilibrium.

- The parents found some stability from the relief of tension.
- The solidarity of the family was, to all intents and purposes, maintained.
- The family problems and their disruptive potential were held in check.

The following dysfunctional factors occurred:

- Disturbing secondary complications developed.
- Extra realistic tasks and problems were generated for the family.
- The victim developed a potential to fight back.

- The victim started to have increasing problems outside the family.
- Because of the functional factors of the process it can continue for a very long time and thus cause serious disturbance to the victim.

Discussion

Some of the causes of tension noted here are unique to the kind of multi-ethnic society examined, but the issue of *tension-creation*, however it arises, is fundamental to the process of family scapegoating. Such tensions form the basis of the power, the energy which is essential to drive the family members into the process of trying to find some way within the existing boundaries to relieve the pressure. The net result, as we have seen, is that the blame is transferred onto some member of the family.

The other very large issues which have implications for scapegoating in clearly defined group situations are, first, the *external factors* which force the group to find the solutions to its problems within its own boundaries and, second, the *guilt* which arises in the scapegoaters about their ambivalent attitudes to the victim they have unwittingly created. This latter factor tends to be split between despair and anger at the behaviour of the victim and tacit encouragement and the giving of indirect reward for exactly that same behaviour.

Other points worthy of note are the *symbolic nature* of the choice of victim and the possibility that choice is also founded upon *obvious difference* and, finally, because of the probable long-term nature of the process, the considerable damage which accrues to the child scapegoat. The long-term nature of the process is dictated by the fact that the process actually works, and this must cause concern because (a) the question of ultimate cost has to be addressed and (b) if any attempt at intervention is contemplated, it is not just the process that has to be replaced but also its success in relieving the tension. There is no doubt that, in the case of family scapegoating, success occurs when a state of balance is reached but it must never be forgotten that this is only achieved at a high cost to the victim.

SCAPEGOATING IN ORGANISATIONS

In 1964 Heap described the behaviour of a group of 14/15-year-olds who were members of a youth club which contained two hostile subgroups: one was boisterous, rough and 'highly excitable', the other was more controlled and more decorous in its behaviour. Between the two groups were several club members who were committed to neither group but had access to both and were thus not isloated. One girl, Elisabeth, aged 15½, was sexually promiscuous and flaunted her behaviour and style of provocative dressing. She was also regarded by all the other members, who had virtually no contact with the opposite sex, as having very low standards and they condemned her behaviour especially in relation to their own 'respectable' conduct.

Heap relates how the girls in this group not only had normal adolescent problems relating to curiosity and sexual wishes, but they also had members who had been subjected to sexual assault. Others had brutal parents and divorced parents with adultery as the main cause. He says, 'Their sexual fantasies would thus be exceptionally loaded with guilt and fear, since their experience and observation had been that to surrender to sexual impulse is highly destructive, that sex is in every sense "bad"!'

So Elisabeth became the focus of the group's projected sexuality and was punished by them, both for acting out for the group and for actually doing so.

However, there was another side to this behaviour: Elisabeth had complex and difficult problems of her own in relation to her family background, and becoming the focal point of the group's hostility provided her with some attention which she could otherwise never have received. Her behaviour was therefore deliberately provocative and in this respect she could fulfil some of her own deep needs.

Elisabeth's role as scapegoat was most clearly demonstrated when she was temporarily removed from the group by being taken into care because of a deteriorating home situation. The group was then compelled to discover other ways of dealing with their concepts of sexuality and 'badness', and this was achieved through using the offices of an understanding social worker. It is most interesting to note that when Elisabeth returned to the group after her enforced absence the group had resolved some of the problems that had compelled them to make her the scapegoat and treated her with much more compassion. As a consequence, her provocative behaviour noticeably diminished.

Heap did not tell us whether this change in her role within the group actually rendered Elisabeth more dissatisfied with her membership. For the other side of the scapegoat equation in her case was that her needs were being met by the process just as much as those of the group. Although the pressure to keep the problems within the bounds of the group are not as strong in an organisation like a youth club as they are in a family with its very intense loyalties, the nature of the adolescents' problems meant that some degree of secrecy must have been present. Given that all the factors of choice were there within the group, and that they coincided to a great degree with the needs of the group, then some form of scapegoating was almost inevitable.

Another and somewhat similar scapegoating situation in a youth club is described by Gisela Konopka (1963: 57):

The rejected isolate sometimes becomes the scapegoat of the group. He is not rejected for something he is himself, but something the group projects on him – group projection frequently being as unconscious as individual projection.

The situation of the rejected isolate and subsequent scapegoating is so irrational and based upon unconscious motivation that it produces a situation that is uncommonly difficult to work with, as we shall see later in Chapters 9 and 10. Konopka gives, as an example, the situation of a 14/15-year-old girl, Carol, who was under constant attack by her club member peers because they perceived her as a 'bad girl' and 'oversexed'. The other girls in the group were very anxious about sex and Carol had a mature physical appearance.

Once more there is no indication of what the girls actually thought at the time they attacked Carol, but there is an assumption on the part of the worker that they were experiencing anxieties, fears and guilt about their own sexuality which were projected onto Carol. This, it was assumed, would give them both the opportunity to punish Carol for being what they secretly longed to be themselves, and at the same time to distance themselves from Carol. There is some suggestion in this analysis that the distancing factor gives vicarious pleasure – i.e. it allows one to watch someone being or doing something which appears desirable but is forbidden and also offers the freedom to dissociate oneself from such behaviour and to disown one's own desires. In essence, enjoying vicarious pleasure in the forbidden while still remaining in one's own eyes relatively pure.

Another example, this time from an industrial situation, is given by Coch and French (1948: 326–7). They describe a cohesive subgroup in the workplace that set a standard concerning production, 'Where the attitudes toward management are antagonistic, this group standard may take the form of a definite restriction of production to a given level.' These authors add that this was especially the case when, by being transferred to a new job, the group were set a new piece rate. By setting their own level of production at a lower rate the group believed that they would force the rate to be altered in their favour if it seemed that they could not achieve the set rate.

Into this group came a person with a different attitude to the work in hand and who, as a result, started to produce at a rate that was considerably higher than the one established by the group as their informal norm. Within a very short space of time the new worker became the scapegoat of the group. Indeed, the authors give a summary of the units of work produced and show the stage at which such scapegoating began. Where the average rate of the group was 50 units per hour, by day 4 the new man had already passed this level. By day 12 he was 6 units above the level and the researchers noted that at this stage scapegoating began. The new man's rate then began to drop until another transfer occurred and he became a single worker with no group standard to maintain. At this stage his work rate almost doubled in the next 20 days. The authors noted that most of the characteristics of scapegoating were present in this incident. The workers were incensed at the management for setting a level which they considered too high but which they could not challenge directly for fear of losing their jobs. There was also dislike of the new man; he was close to the other workers and he demonstrated a great and obvious difference in his attitude to work performance. The aggression that could not be expressed was thus directed quite specifically at the new worker.

This example shows quite clearly that a difference, in this case a difference of attitude, can be virtually anything at all. The new worker in this example had not had time to adjust to the ideas of his colleagues and his difference was one that they believed could destroy their ability to try to sabotage what they considered to be an excessive rate for the job.

SCAPEGOATING IN SMALL GROUPS

Consequently the hypothesis now is that Al is 'selected' as scapegoat because she exemplifies those traits perceived as 'bad' by the consultant. It seems to members that the consultant desires them not to have these traits.

They avoid being deemed the possessors of undesirable traits by locating them in one person. (Organisational defence against persecution anxiety.)

(Long 1992: 150)

This brief analysis of the reason for Al being scapegoated arises from the records of a group lasting for fourteen sessions designed for members to explore the processes and dynamics arising within the group as they happened.

In session 6 Al came under direct attack, but the records showed that it was the culmination of a long process of building tension. Al was the subject of the group's anger because she evaded discussing her feelings with the group and because of other 'annoying' habits. These included the kind of language she used.

Long eventually suggests that Al became a scapegoat because:

She focussed the anger felt by members at perceived attacks on their own traits or behaviour which by projection became hers alone.

She was believed to be the focus of the consultant's anger at the group and on many occasions she was seen to be holding the group back.

(1992: 151–2)

Indeed the group may have deeply resented the consultant's attitude to them, but believing her to be all powerful they attacked A1 instead when her behaviour suggested that she was vulnerable.

A good example of the scapegoating process in a therapeutic group is given by F. Kraupl-Taylor in an article in *New Society* in 1964. The group comprised young women selected on the basis that they all had in common 'neurotic anxiety and self-consciousness'. All except one of the group had led reputable lives with no transgressions of the existing moral code. The one who was different had engaged in several casual sexual relationships about which she felt guilty. For this reason she was definitely regarded as a low status member of the group and contributed little to the group's discussions.

However, as the group approached the treatment stage that required them to reveal the conflict between their sexual desires and their fears, some role-play started in a fairly innocuous way outside of the group. As these ventures faded into failure, the group looked upon the one member with sexual experience as knowledgeable and pressurised her into a sexual relationship with a casual acquaintance, about which she felt very guilty. Now the group could really crucify her for her immoral behaviour, despite the fact that they were probably aware that she had acted in a sense on their behalf. Their pious condemnation provoked their victim into roundly condemning them for their hypocrisy, with the end result that a more free and open discussion of their sexual difficulties was possible through an examination, initially, of the processes and manoeuvres of the group.

Most of the characteristics that define the scapegoating process are represented in this episode. The group were approaching a point in their treatment when self-exposure would be required and would include a revelation of their fears, mainly of a sexual nature. They were thus becoming increasingly aware of what might be called their collective 'badness', and because this was uncomfortable they searched for ways in which, with minimal cost to themselves, they could discharge this badness. There was one member in the group who was different in that the others knew she had in the past behaved in ways which they would describe as amoral. In addition to this, she was held in very low esteem.

Although they were curious about her experiences, they appeared to have no way of taking advantage of this; however, they could offload their 'badness' onto her symbolically, and when she actually performed in the way they desired of her, they punished her by excoriating her behaviour. Indeed, in earlier times they would have driven her out for her wickedness, making her carry their wickedness with her as well.

However, in this instance they had misjudged the nature of their scapegoat. In the classic form the scapegoat should have been either a willing volunteer in the process or too weak and too powerless to resist. In this case she was neither, and, resenting her 'victim' role and powered by her sense of injustice and self-guilt, she exposed the hypocrisy of the scapegoat gambit. This, fortunately, led to a more open and frank discussion of the problems involved through an analysis of the scapegoating process. It could have been a far less beneficial outcome if the group had been less prepared to enter into discussion of their behaviour. Indeed, head-on confrontation could just as easily have been the result.

Taylor does not make clear what the group thought they were doing when they 'set up' their scapegoat or how they justified to themselves the subsequent behaviour. Such an analysis was not an essential part of his article. Although the behaviour of the group – with the solitary exception of their wrong assessment of the powerlessness of their victim – followed the classic scapegoating procedure, this fact cannot have occurred to them until the process was later explained through discussion. So what did they think they were doing?

Usually when groups are asked to discuss some process they have recently survived, some emphasis is placed upon the almost universal dislike of the victim and disgust at their behaviour, but even more emphasis is placed upon the obvious differences which, over time, have been revealed and recognised in the group. However, there is very little in the literature which actually compares the thoughts and beliefs of those who have gone through the process of scapegoating either as victim or scapegoater.

Summary

It remains now only to summarise some of the points that have been demonstrated by the above examples.

Maintenance

Most of the examples show that the members of the groups concerned had some clear idea that unless something was done their groups were going to be in substantial difficulties. What they chose to do, if 'chose' is the right word, was to scapegoat a member of the group and expect that person to bear the blame for all that was going wrong.

Difference

This appears to be the main way in which the member who became the scapegoat was selected. It is interesting to speculate that if the problems had been different in the groups just studied, would the members chosen to be scapegoats have been the same? All smallish groups have, as a natural feature, the high degree of visibility of their members so that any differences are immediately noticeable, and thus factors such as low status and deviant behaviour are attention-drawing when the group is looking for someone to blame. The industrial group showed that difference does not necessarily have to be something worse than what is considered to be 'normal', but could be something better – in this case, a higher standard of work performance.

Congruence

The fit between the difference of the potential scapegoat's behaviour and the group's current problem is worth noting. In several of the examples the person selected as scapegoat had behaviour patterns which coincided very closely with areas of immense interest to the other group members, but which they were forbidden to indulge in by virtue of external or internal prohibition.

Scapegoat's needs

The most effective and at the same time devastating scapegoating procedures occurred when the process not only met the needs of the group but also some of the needs of the victim. Certainly those needs, mainly for attention of some sort, added double the power to the process. Perhaps the victim, if given a choice, would not have chosen to gain some relief of his or her needs in exactly this way, but it is most likely that he or she had discovered in the past no other successful gambit. As one author put it about the family scapegoat:

> He or she is the member of the family who is deemed to be the one in need of help and brought to the agency as the one in trouble. Often he is the scapegoated one who is described as the most difficult, disturbed, disruptive member of the family.
> (Whiffen 1978: 158)

The point being made is that once the scapegoat is in this position he or she cannot be dislodged from it because it is the only position he or she has.

Boundaries

This point has already been covered but it does little harm to restate it here. Families and small groups do have bonds and loyalties and are quite well aware in most cases that what goes on within the group is the group's private business. Such need to confine activities, especially those which the group regards with some degree of alarm or shame, puts a limitation on the number of individuals who are available to be scapegoated.

The family victim

The favourite role for the family scapegoat appears to be that of the patient or the 'sick one'.

> The most common example of such alienation is the family scapegoat process, whereby one family member is identified as the 'patient', the 'sick one', the one for whom the family seek therapy. This person is often the one who is most different or *apart* from family norms or 'rules'. In Gestalt terms, this individual may be seen as the 'disowned' or 'projected' part of the family system.
>
> (Campbell 1973: 78–9)

Lack of alternatives

In one sense this is caused by the bonds referred to in the item 'Boundaries' above, but it is also clear that to blame someone for what is happening often seems like the only available action without also increasing the danger too much.

Fundamental urge

Most of the examples show that, irrespective of the level at which the process occurs, what lies behind it is some fundamental urge to escape from the pressures of being held responsible for bad feelings and events.

Vicarious pleasure

Where the scapegoat was performing an act that was forbidden in some way to the other members of the group, then one of the driving forces behind the compulsion to perform was the fact that the members derived pleasure from seeing someone do something they wanted to do but could not.

Groups can become scapegoats

It must be stated that scapegoats are not necessarily single individuals. In large organisations containing many small groups, these small groups play the same part *vis-à-vis* the containing organisation that an individual plays with regard to the small group of which he or she is a member.

CONCLUSION

The recorded examples that have been given here and elsewhere throughout this book are representative of the process of scapegoating in the family, in organisations and in small groups. The supposition that the problems which produced this process were of a particular nature – e.g. the sexual problems of young people which may be regarded as pertaining to the time in which they were recorded and thus no longer relevant – is fallacious. Problems change from generation to generation and from place to place. But the essential point is that the response pattern, the basic moves of the process of scapegoating, are exactly the same whatever kind of problem forms the basis of the essential energy that drives the search for relief.

One point that I shall take up again in Chapter 11 concerns the apparent general increase in the willingness to blame which seems to have developed in our society over approximately the last thirty years. It would appear that there is a strong and perhaps developing belief that our problems are inevitably the fault of someone other than ourselves. To blame the government, indeed any decision-making body or individual, is always the first option rather than some consideration by the individual that he or she may actually be mainly responsible for what has happened.

Thus, an enormous increase in the cry 'Scapegoat' has occurred over the last few years, which obviously derives from a growing climate of opinion supporting the idea that all difficulties and problems are essentially the fault of others, of mismanagement or of inadequate care. This is not to say that others are *not* responsible for some of our problems; quite the contrary. But it is evident that the burden of responsibility, or an increasing proportion of it, is being laid at the doors of others. This is accompanied by a growing suspicion that a considerable part of this increase is due to a general opinion that evasion and the transfer of blame to others, whether responsible or not, is an entirely appropriate and approved action.

The examples of family scapegoating given here stress the limitation of choice of scapegoat based on the bonds existing within the family group. There is much discussion about the family currently and it may well be that the bonding pressures are less than they were and thus also less often the basis of choice of scapegoat. Their place may have been taken by the pressures of the immediate community in which family groups live.

Chapter 6

Victims
Examples of victimisation

Throughout history the dominant majority has sought out and punished scapegoats. If the age-old idea of the scapegoat were true and we really could cure some of the ills of our society by sacrificing a few individuals, there might be something to be said for it and the only difficulty would be to decide who is to be next. But the sacrifice does not decrease our troubles. It increases them. Not only is it unjust and cruel to the goat, it covers up the problems instead of solving them. The scapegoat's punishment deflects the same fate from us for the sins we have committed ourselves. At the same time the scapegoat provides us with the flattering illusion that we are superior to him. . . . In recent years the user of cannabis has been used as a convenient scapegoat and has been persecuted with a vindictiveness that is not related to the harm he has caused, but rather to the mythical magnitude of his wickedness.

(Schofield 1971: 178–9)

For an article in the *Daily Telegraph* of Saturday, 16 June 1992, David Crane produced the following title, 'How could Helen spend those years with a wimp like Paris? Menelaus has red hair!' Bright and snappy as the title is, and with good humorous content, it highlights one of the most interesting factors of the process of scapegoating which concerns the ways in which victims are chosen or emerge. When victims are chosen, as our survey of ancient practices has shown, that choice rests upon the perception of some clearly definable and observable difference of the proposed victim to his or her selectors. David Crane chose to write about one such obvious difference – red hair.

Stated as baldly as that it appears ridiculous that the fate of an individual should depend upon the colour of his or her hair. But, nevertheless, when victims have to be found to be sacrificed in some way then such significant and visible differences are to be discovered in the lists of possible candidates held in mind by the scapegoaters.

> If I should ever be called upon to act professionally, I am happy to think that there will be no difficulty in finding plenty of people whose loss will be a distinct gain to society at large.

Thus says Ko-Ko, expatiating on his role as Lord High Executioner in *The Mikado*. The song that follows starts thus:

> As some day it may happen that a victim must be found,
> I've got a little list – I've got a little list
> Of society offenders who might well be underground,
> And who never would be missed – who never would be missed!
>   (W.S. Gilbert 1885)

The song continues to detail those whose behaviour – offensive, irritating and always extremely visible – marks them out as potential victims. In truth, none of those listed would actually have committed a crime that merited summary execution as an appropriate punishment. They would become sacrificial victims so that Ko-Ko could maintain his status and conform to the laws of the Mikado, and they would be chosen on the basis of possessing purely irritating and visible habits.

I am sure that Gilbert knew well enough that, humorous as this song is, it was likely to ring all kinds of bells in the minds of his audiences who almost to an individual would have experienced in their own lives the substitution and victimisation thesis he was propounding.

Of course we live surrounded by extremely visible differences in people every day of our lives, and while such differences as red hair or irritating behaviour may focus our attention they are surely wholly inadequate as a basis for selecting a possible victim. There must be some other factor. Indeed, there are many other factors, of which four will serve to illustrate our point: extreme dislike, fear, ignorance and the displacement of blame from powerful originators to those perceived to be much weaker. It is also to be noted that, as Gilbert inferred, many of the factors involved in victim selection are related to prejudice, often of a highly personal kind.

Historically, incidents of substitution occur when the individual really at fault was considered to be of too high a status to receive punishment. These are quite simply examples of victimisation – but not, I hasten to add, in the modern sense of the word because it is usually quite obvious that the 'victims' in these historical examples believed as strongly in the rightness of what they were asked to do as those who imposed the function upon them.

The Oxford dictionary defines victim as: 'Living being sacrificed to a deity or in performance of a religious rite; person, thing, injured or destroyed in pursuit of an object; in gratification of a passion, etc., or as a result of event or circumstance.' This chapter is about victims; it provides examples of modern scapegoats and attempts to analyse both how they become victims and what the consequences frequently are.

In 1930 Daphne du Maurier wrote a novel with the title *The Scapegoat*. The plot involved an English lecturer on holiday in France who was the identical physical counterpart of a French nobleman who was in considerable difficulty both financially and also in terms of his relationships. The plot tells how the lecturer, without his consent, is substituted for the nobleman so that the latter can murder his wife and inherit her fortune to pay off his debts, leaving the lecturer to accept the blame or to provide an alibi by being somewhere else when the crime was committed. In either case he would then become disposable.

This story can serve as a fairly clear example of one of the major differences between the modern concept of the scapegoat and that of the ancients. In the du Maurier story the lecturer is framed deliberately and with malicious intent, not to assuage the anger of the gods but precisely to become a cover, which can be eliminated later, for the acts of another. Admittedly, the cover might have been expected to suffer the consequences of those acts even to the elimination process being performed as an act of judicial execution. But the major thrust of the plot is the deliberate attempt of one individual to force an unwilling other to hide the former's misdoings and, if necessary, suffer the consequences attendant upon them. Thus du Maurier's scapegoat is much closer to the concept of the whipping boy than to that of the biblical scapegoat. Not only have the reasons for scapegoating changed in their emphasis but so also have the form of choosing the victim and, more importantly, the expected outcomes. In this chapter we shall consider the reasons that form the basis of the motivation for the act of scapegoating. The choice of victim, the process of scapegoating and the expected outcomes shall be considered subsequently.

In 1992 Paddy Ashdown, leader of the Liberal Democrat party, was forced to declare publicly that he had had an affair with his secretary some five years earlier, because a document detailing this behaviour sequence – which had been prepared by Ashdown's solicitor in view of the fact that the secretary was filing for divorce – had been stolen from the solicitor's office and offered to the press. The letter was not the only thing stolen but the fact that it was offered to the press for a substantial sum of money indicated that whoever stole it knew that it had a blackmail value.

Mr Ashdown admitted publicly that the affair had occurred. His admission was accepted by most of his colleagues and by the general public as the correct behaviour of an honourable man. Indeed, shortly afterwards the polls showed that his personal rating, and that of his party, had increased. His personal behaviour could have adversely affected his party's interests. If the poll rating had gone down there is every indication that he would have been blamed. He would have been made a scapegoat.

People in the public eye are often scapegoated in the modern sense for behaviour which, while relatively common among others, can be used by public agencies as an excuse for their failure to win or maintain public approval when, in fact, that lack of approval can be accredited to actual failure of performance.

The ancients, as we have seen in Chapter 3, believed that their everyday behaviour was supervised by gods and that incorrect behaviour was visited with punishment. Because the link between cause and effect was not clearly understood, it must have seemed that such a situation was the only logical answer to the question of how acts performed in secrecy were known about and punished. For this reason they indulged in acts of propitiation, requests for forgiveness and the presentation of acceptable gifts to the gods. All significantly religious communities and individuals maintain this belief in some form or other. In essence, what has just been described could be stated quite simply as a system for the evasion of consequence.

For example, when Prometheus brought fire down to earth for the benefit of mankind he was punished by being chained to a rock where a raven continually pecked at his vitals. He had defied the gods. Now it is only possible to defy something that you actually believe exists. In this myth, the purpose of which was to instruct ordinary mortals of what would happen to them if they did not conform to the accepted way of life, Prometheus is depicted as one who knew the possible consequences of his action but was prepared to take the risk, believing that it was justifiable.

There are many factors here that we must now pursue in some detail. For instance, I have said that the ancients did not seem to have a very clear idea of the laws of cause and effect, but do modern people have any better idea? Admittedly, they seldom seem to be inclined to place the blame for their problems onto supernatural agencies, although it is relevant to mention that something called luck or fate is still considered to be a contributing factor. Nevertheless, it is still possible to find people who see a connection between their walking out of their front door and it starting to rain. This is a teleological fallacy, but events that occur in sequence are very frequently linked in the sense that those occurring first are supposed to have intitiated those occurring later.

If we no longer believe that we are being continuously watched, supervised and monitored by supernatural beings, then why do we still feel it necessary to take steps to evade consequences? There are, perhaps, only two possible answers to this question: public image and conscience. Before examining these two factors, however, let us return to the central theme of consequence.

Freud informed the world that all behaviour was purposive. He was not the first person to say this but he made his statement at a time when it was possible for its impact to be very widespread. What he meant in very simple terms was that all human behaviour, whether conscious, unconscious, instinctive or abnormal, was brought into being by a perception that circumstances existed which demanded a response. Behaviour occurs in order to achieve something.

While this is obviously true, it is insufficient to leave the statement unqualified. Alongside it we have to put the *fact* of consequence. All behaviour produces consequences, but they have to be seen in the context of time. An inescapable conclusion of everyday life is that behaviour produced as a response to perceived circumstances also produces unforeseen effects that have a habit of being much more important that the goal of the original response. The classical illustration of the process of displacement may be used as an example.

A man at work is given a bad time by his boss which makes him both very angry and very frustrated. He is angry because he has been treated so cavalierly and he is frustrated because he believes there is nothing he can do about it. His boss is powerful. The man has many responsibilities which are dependent for their fulfilment upon his maintaining himself in employment. He cannot, therefore, vent his anger on the cause of it. He is afraid of the consequences. However, when he returns to his office there is a subordinate who is not a person who poses the same risk for he, too, is in the position of being dependent. And so the subordinate receives the anger generated by the boss. The tale goes on through layers of people, all of whom accept anger they did not cause for the simple reason that to do otherwise would pose unacceptable risks.

There are several points to be made from the above passage. First, the boss's response was, as far as he was concerned, dictated by the situation as he saw it. He had an end in view and obviously achieved it. What he did not foresee was all the ensuing consequences. These, indeed, may have been far wider than was related here, since all of the people concerned would have taken the effect of the encounter they had into other aspects of their lives whether immediately or at some time in the future. This leads to the next point to be explored.

When our responses to situations are conscious – that is, intended or planned – they have the qualities of being inevitably based on three factors. They are based, first, upon the amount and quality of knowledge about the situation that is available to us at the time; second, upon our previous experience of similar situations; and third, upon the amount of time we believe is available to make the response. Part of this information pack is our perception of the possible consequences of what we propose to do, i.e. the risk factor.

Now the fact is quite simply that this information pack is limited in scope and is also frequently inaccurate. Consequences which arise later and have to be evaded cause many people to say that the major effects of any social action might well be those that are never foreseen in the original plan. That this sort of situation puts individuals into the position of having to make a response – as we shall see later when they are accused of doing something which others affected by their action regard as detrimental – often provides the initial impetus for an action which is largely a matter of transferring the blame onto someone else. Unexpected consequences are often the basic cause of scapegoating, especially when the people involved are public figures.

In June 1992, Mr Kinnock was reported as appealing to the Labour Party to address the fundamental causes of its election defeat and to refrain from squabbling over campaign mistakes or searching for scapegoats.

In public life the allocation of blame for the palpable failure of an organisation to achieve its avowed goals, frequently takes the form mentioned above. Someone has to be placed in the situation of accepting, or at least of being accused of, responsibility for the débâcle. The major problem is that in such large-scale organisations as the Labour Party, the possible reasons for failure are seldom clearly defined, almost never simple or single and are always and inevitably subject to various opinions and backed by various authorities. In the example given, the Labour Party have variously suggested that failure to be elected was a result of (i) the way the public regarded the party's economic proposals, (ii) the triumphalism of the last days of the campaign, (iii) the perception of the party as belonging to the past and having outdated ideas, (iv) the perception that the party stifled enterprise, (v) the personality of the then leader Neil Kinnock, (vi) the biased and deviant reporting of Labour's policy by sections of the press, (vii) the memory of past Labour administrations, etc.

The point is not that any or all of these defined causes are necessarily untrue, but that there are so many of them, and beyond saying that they are all partially responsible for what happened, or until some more objective, dispassionate and neutral investigation is done, what remains is opinion.

Of course this is not all. What also exists is a considerable amount of frustration, disappointment, bitterness, anger and hurt and these are the emotional factors that tend to colour the initial search for the reason for failure and very quickly to attribute maximum blame in selected quarters.

It is in this highly charged, emotional atmosphere that victims are selected, and certain people are set up to carry the blame. Once a victim has been exposed and pilloried, then a cathartic effect is produced and the members of the organisation have temporarily cleansed themselves of the frustration brought about by the failure.

Unfortunately, because of the illogicality that usually accompanies the choice of scapegoats in such circumstances, a considerable amount of injustice is usually involved which sows the seeds within the organisation of probable strife at some later date.

If we look more closely at the actions of an organisation in these circumstances, we are likely to discover that some selected person(s) is/are being sacrificed to allow the organisation to maintain some level of functional efficiency. Sometimes deals are struck along the lines of the victim being compensated for accepting the scapegoat role, where some balance may be established between what the victim will lose by this action, e.g. prestige, promotion, job, etc., and what advantage can be gained, e.g. freedom to look elsewhere, to change allegiance, etc.

Essentially the victims are chosen, as are all scapegoats who are not self-selected, on the criteria we have already discussed, viz.: in the opinion of the majority, they are dispensable; their sacrifice will suffice to effect a face-saving solution that will contain the elements of survival and at not too great a cost to the organisation; the selected victims will undoubtedly possess visible attributes which have in the past been a source of irritation to their colleagues; and, finally, their excision from the organisation will produce rather more benefit than disaster.

Once these factors have been concluded, and the victims chosen and expelled, then the organisation will have succeeded in despatching with those victims the blame for the failure that occurred. This is the classic scapegoat procedure. In the past, those involved in the ritual of scapegoating invariably regarded it as a religious rite and also believed implicitly in the fact that evil was tangible and could be transferred, but in modern public life no such beliefs exist. In the ancient rituals the scapegoat was truly sacrificed, i.e. he or she was usually killed. In modern sacrifices the victim is not very often eliminated in this final sense and so a relatively new phenomenon emerges, which is that of the scapegoat, some time after victimisation, seeking redress for wrongful dismissal, punishment, etc. Indeed, latterly we have witnessed people who were sent to prison for crimes which subsequent investigation has demonstrated that either they did not commit or there was insufficient evidence to prove that they did.

Why did such apparent miscarriages of justice take place? The answer may be quite simple.

Most of the offences for which these people were imprisoned concerned acts of violence, and were frequently decribed as acts of terrorism. Public opinion – which has become more apathetic over many years of exposure to such events – has, in the past been extremely horrified by acts of wanton murder of innocent people and thus public pressure has been enormous on the police and law enforcement agencies to discover the perpetrators and bring them to justice. To discover such terrorists may be relatively easy but to find sufficient irrefutable evidence of their involvement in a particular incident is not. Thus people are selected to become victims by use of the same criteria that, as we have noted, are used in all cases of scapegoating.

It is essential to point out that, like the majority of scapegoating activities, these imprisonments were entirely successful in assuaging public demands for punishment, but not those of the victims' immediate relatives and friends. When, years later, the victims are found to have been innocent, public attitudes change and the release of the victims tends to be met with little condemnation and some sense that justice has at last been done. But this has two corollaries: (1) if these people are innocent of the crimes for which they were sentenced, then who actually committed them?; (2) *if* the process was one of scapegoating, then the public tend to regard those who initiated this process as being violators of natural justice and there is a demand that those responsible should be found and punished.

Thus one clear distinction emerges among several between the modern practice of public scapegoating and that practised long ago. The former tends to produce a self-perpetuating process, since driving the scapegoat out is *not* a final solution which culminates in the victim's death. Modern victims remain in existence, and sometimes fight against the personal injustice they suffered.

There are two points about the act of scapegoating which can be derived from the actions of the Labour Party following their election defeat. One may be called the process of counter-scapegoating, and the second concerns the self-selecting victim.

Counter-scapegoating behaviour is a modern situation in that it is dependent for its existence on two factors. First, the scapegoat is no longer killed and, second, there are usually several people in positions that carry some of the responsibility for ordering the organisation's affairs. This is part of the complicated system of responsibility which, in most cases, is primarily responsible for the problem of allocating blame. When such an organisation is in the early stages of a review of failure, it is looking for reasons and there is a plethora of possibilities. Counter-scapegoating arises because all of the individuals in positions of possible blame are wholly aware of their vulnerability to accusation. Their response is almost to make public their accusation of others within the system. This counter- or sometimes pre-emptive accusation immediately muddies the waters, but it also has the effect of diminishing the possibility of the accuser being held solely responsible for what has occurred.

The request by Mr Kinnock that his party should cease looking for scapegoats was a direct reference to such acts of counter-scapegoating that were taking place.

The process was even further complicated and motivations multiplied by the fact that, as leader of the party, Mr Kinnock resigned, thus symbolically drawing to himself the responsibility for his party's failure. This is traditional practice and no one is compelled to accept that such a self-sacrifice actually means that the person concerned believes that he or she was solely responsible for what happened. Tradition has, however, shown that one of the responsibilities of leadership is to accept symbolic responsibility for failure, so that the search for whoever or whatever may have been truly responsible does not destroy the public image of the organisation.

However, the complicating factor that Mr Kinnock's resignation produced was the necessity for the party to elect a new leader and deputy. This process is one where potential candidates attempt to gain backing for their nomination within the party, and thus there is a clear need to project an electable image. The obverse of this process is, of course, to highlight the unelectable side of any opposing candidates. In the case we are reviewing it became obvious that one of the major factors that could render a candidate relatively unelectable was to show that the candidate had been largely responsible for the election failure.

The behaviour of politicians is no different in kind from that of all members of organisations when they face a public which has strong evidence of failure. A combination of the need to preserve the structure of the organisation, at least as a form of public image, and to ensure the survival of the major actors in the drama, dictates that sacrifices have to be made. And lest we think that the modern form of scapegoating which eschews execution is less horrific than the classical version, it must be noted that some scapegoats have indeed been executed until relatively recently and such an ending may still be occurring in some parts of the world. However, with disgrace, humiliation, dismissal and exile, which are the more usual forms of modern practice in public life, it can be said that the process of scapegoating has retained a considerable amount of its ability to destroy its victims, and the basic facts of how such victims are chosen remains the same.

FAMILY VICTIMS

The characteristics of victims found in the process of scapegoating within the family comprise a very interesting and wide-ranging study. Once it becomes possible to distinguish between those characteristics and behaviours that existed prior to victimisation from those that develop or are enhanced after it, virtually anything that can call attention to an individual seems to serve as a cause for selection.

For instance, the way in which an individual responds to the charges and accusations that are common in family life appears to be sufficient.

> Everyone began by blaming Sandra, who at first appeared to seek acceptance, then became stubborn and defensive, eventually wept and finally did in the group *what she was always said to do at home* – excluded herself. . . .
>
> (Skynner 1971c: 4)

As Skynner goes on to tell us, this stubborn refusal to accept blame for her behaviour, which included stealing, jealousy and being provocative, meant that Sandra 'had been driven relentlessly into opposition'. Her parents and her siblings reported that by her behaviour she had generated intense frustration in her father and a sense of helplessness and inadequacy in her mother.

Sandra was the second child in a family of five; her older sister, her senior by one year, Susan, appeared to represent all that the family required of a child. She was well behaved, conforming and an achiever. It is interesting to speculate that the choice of Sandra as scapegoat may have rested initially almost entirely on the fact that she was different from Susan. No doubt the tensions which existed within the family would have needed a point of discharge somewhere within in it, but Sandra's comparison with Susan and the immediate disappointment this aroused might well have been the most important selection factor. This is backed by the fact that other children in the family group were younger and more vulnerable than Sandra, and thus probably weaker in terms of defending themselves. But Sandra's story demonstrates that being chosen as a scapegoat when the need arises can depend not upon the more obvious and solid differences of characteristics and provocative behaviour but upon something as simple as not living up to expectations set by another and earlier member of the family.

Skynner (1971b: 10) presented another scapegoat victim, Pam, a girl of 14. Her behaviour on referral included being destructive, being hostile to her mother, depression, separation-anxiety, stealing, truanting and sexual acting out. She presented as controlled, sitting clumsily slumped in her chair.

Once again there was an older sister, Sarah, who was 17, calm, self-possessed and an obvious comparison. She was also the recipient of much family praise. The selection process here may just have been that Pam was the second child. Sarah, the first born, had been 'the receptacle into which all the family's good qualities were projected for safe keeping'. Given the facts that the tensions in the family grew rather than that they were dispersed, that Sarah's role as repository of good feelings was already well established and, finally, that there was as always a strong need to deal with the problems within the context of the family group, the only possible victim was Pam!

The essential basis of the selection of Pam as the family scapegoat rested on the fact that no one else within the family was available. The restrictive factor in the family group usually seems to be the necessity of keeping the tension and the conflict within the bounds of the group. Whether this is based upon a sense of loyalty or a sense of guilt or just on the belief that the family's problems belong to them and to no one else is difficult to define. But the same pattern of 'keep it within the group' tends to emerge in other groups but without the strong relationships and dependencies that exist within a family.

The selection having been made, the tension of fulfilling the role then tends to generate behaviour patterns in the victim which amply justify the group's choice, as witness the catalogue of behaviours with which Pam presented upon referral.

VICTIMS IN ORGANISATIONS

Scapegoating in an organisation demonstrates some of the same processes as in groups. Inevitably the selection of the scapegoat, whether it is a small group within the organisation or an individual, depends to a large extent upon a perception of possibility. For instance, because organisations tend to be larger than groups – indeed, are often a multi-group system – then selection of a scapegoat to take the blame for what is apparently wrong with the organisation always seems to be rational to the extent that the victim(s) are credible responsible agents who could actually be the cause of the difficulties. Inevitably the prime target element is the management structure or some selected part of it, but however large or small the element selected, it must be able to be seen as potentially capable of creating the problems.

Organisational scapegoating has one great similarity to the same process in smaller groups in that although there is tension and conflict within the system – and most individuals within that system are aware of this and find it more or less intolerable – the actual sources of that tension are not clearly known. Indeed, given the complexity of the system, the many variable and different agendas it contains, and the diversity of contact all subsumed under pursuit of the system's general goals, then it is not surprising that the location of the causes of tension and conflict should not only be inaccurately assessed but also disparate.

Nevertheless, tension needs to be discharged and blame allocated, so while difference once again plays a large part, availability and perceived potential also come into focus, as can be seen in the following example.

A hospice, which had been in operation for several years and was well regarded for the quality of its work, developed what appeared to be minor areas of conflict and disagreement between different levels of staff, between staff and committee, between the volunteers and others. Gradually it dawned on various individuals that the number of complaints, conflicts and difficulties was rapidly growing and, moreover, that problems apparently stemming from a wide diversity of people and areas within the system were beginning to coalesce around the administrative central person, the matron. This process reached a climax when different parts of the system began to make requests that the matron should be replaced, averring that she was responsible for an enormous variety of ills ranging from some small mishandling of drugs to the conduct of individuals.

Matron was being scapegoated.

On investigation, the major factor which generated much of the conflict and tension was found to be simply that, as the hospice had vastly increased the number and quality of its staff and had taken on day care, domiciliary facilities and other responsibilities, the structure of the organisation and of its management had not changed to adapt to or integrate the much larger and more complex functional system. Communications were therefore poor and often misleading, responsibilities were not clearly defined and the sense of being unsupported and unregarded very damaging.

As with the family needing to cope with its own problems within its own boundaries and thus limiting the number of potential scapegoats, the hospice was similarly constrained by the nature of its patients and by an immense professional pride that would not allow personal and work problems to intrude upon their terminally and seriously ill patients. Home life often suffered as a result of trying to resolve tensions there, and fed back in extra resentment into the workplace where it was all discharged upon the one figure who filled all the criteria of being a scapegoat. Matron was different: she was isolated by her role; she did apparently possess the ability to be the essential cause; she was management; and she was an obvious target.

The victim in this case was not a particularly well-liked person and she believed that she was the focus of a personal hate campaign, so that the model became fixed in its parameters until the scapegoat could be driven out. Fortunately, some clarification of the processes was undertaken with outside help and a major readjustment to the management style, based on the increased staffing levels, was set in motion. The beginnings of a support system were thus created.

The major factors in this case were: (a) the conflict and tension arising from a lack of adjustment to growth, which had been hidden in the complexity of a mass of interacting variables but which generated the need to discharge psychic discomfort; (b) the pressure to contain problems and solutions within the system;

and (c) the difference and probable credibility of the selected victim.

The nature of the scapegoat is of particular interest in this case. The factor of difference was represented by three characteristics: the matron was isolated, powerful and disliked. There was also the fact that, like everyone else in the system, she was wholly unaware of the true sources of the conflict and tension and has recorded that she believed the blame laid upon her was a personal vendetta because she had fewer qualifications than some of the senior nursing staff. It did not seem to her that this was a wholly illogical supposition, given the large number of staff and the fact that she knew she had some good longstanding friends. But her responses to what she perceived to be the facts of the situation served only to exacerbate it.

The situation lasted a long time and, like the scapegoats in the families we looked at, both parties – in this case the staff as a whole and matron – became entrapped in their roles. No doubt the process helped the hospice to function and survive, but because nothing was done to remedy the actual causes of conflict the matter had to come to outright confrontation and be resolved with external help.

VICTIMS IN GROUPS

In groups, particularly small groups, one essentially defining characteristic has always been what is casually stated as their 'face-to-face' nature. At the risk of being extremely obvious, but in the interests of clarity, what this means is that each individual member is highly visible, exposed in fact to all the other members of the group for the greater part of the time that the group exists. Indeed, it is an essential factor of small group behaviour that this exposure exists, otherwise the resources which lie ready to be used within the group – the problems and the needs – would never become known and used.

Thus, when it is stated that the main resources of a group are the differences rather than the similarities of the constituent members, the concept of difference needs some further elaboration. Difference offers alternative ways of doing things: alternative attitudes, opinions, thoughts; extra and often unusual approaches, and so on – in effect, differences which are resources or assets because they broaden, deepen and increase possible coping skills, are perfectly acceptable and are indeed essential. But difference can be so different, so irritating and so frustrating that instead of being a positive, adaptable and usable resource it is perceived as a positive hindrance. Some individuals who become scapegoats have developed the art of being different in order to provide for their own needs, then, for a variety of very understandable reasons, have been unable to develop more ordinary and acceptable methods of entering into relationships with others.

A typical example of scapegoating in a small group took place in a half-way house used for individuals being discharged from psychiatric hospital in order that they would be in the community, but still relatively sheltered until they had adapted themselves to that community and were able to live independently within it. A group was held weekly, the members being individuals from both stages of the process – that is, those newly discharged from hospital and those already relocated in the community. In a very long-term sense, it was an open group into which individuals could be admitted as the need for the group's support was discovered. They could then stay as long as that support was required and leave when they felt it was no longer necessary, whether they were residents or not.

The group functioned well in its weekly two-hour meetings, attendance was very regular, contributions were forthcoming from all members and the rather wide variety of backgrounds, ages and experiences produced a large crop of very observable differences, most of which became the bases of learning, experimentation, contacts and increased understanding.

One young man had been socially isolated by his father since the death of his mother when he was very young, and had been kept so, well into his thirties. He had then been admitted to hospital, apparently demonstrating florid mental disturbances when his father died suddenly. He was admitted to the group after a very short stay in hospital. The group, which was largely concerned with relocation into the community after hospitalisation, was considered to be the ideal placement for him. However, what had not been fully assessed was the almost total lack of interactive ability that this otherwise bright young man possessed. All contacts outside the home had been made by his father and the young man's only skills related to being an incarcerated if devoted son. His difference from the others in the group was so great that his behaviour appeared bizarre, but was only really visible as such within the close confines of the group. Their tolerance of this young man's uniquely different behaviour soon wore very thin and they began to believe that he was responsible for their lack of progress. They also believed, and probably rightly, that because he was so different he should not have been placed in their group.

After a few sessions the group turned him into a scapegoat and also the butt of all their own bad feelings about others who frustrated them. Week after week he turned up and was the subject of insult and derision yet made no request to be removed from the group. Often almost in tears at the end of a meeting, he was almost always the first to arrive for the next session. Alternatives were offered and refused. It emerged gradually that although the group were often harsh and cruel, he regarded them as infinitely preferable to the almost totally isolate state in which he had existed. He had been discharged from hospital on the understanding that he would visit the outpatients' clinic and attend the group. The group was a very large part of his small social existence.

Eventually the group were led to see how they were using this willing victim in dealing with their own needs, and were then shown ways of coping with their frustrations with the process of relocation. The young man had never been actively disliked – indeed, most group members had expressed sympathy and his peculiar history was known to them all – but they had all found his difference so frustrating that they had attacked him, and in attacking had found some relief from their own problems at some cost to their victim.

Personalities and situations

Some understanding of the personality and situation of victims in relation to the groups in which they are scapegoated can be obtained from the descriptions of four young scapegoats given by Heap(1964). Indeed, we shall consider these victims again in Chapter 10 when we discuss how their particular situations were dealt with.

Elisabeth

The factors that were instrumental in Elisabeth becoming a scape-goat in a group of fifteen 14–16-year-old girls, members of a large youth club, can be listed as follows:

- Home life – a 'confusion of parental instability, sexual pathology and poverty'.
- Elisabeth – felt worthless, insecure, was sexually promiscuous.
- In-group activity – boastful of her exploits.
- Group response – to give her status and attention.
- Outcome – her needs for attention were met by the scapegoating and the group was able to avoid having to deal with its own problems of growth, identity and sexual development.

As long as Elisabeth was present in the group the members had an ideal way of not facing their own problems, which were brought home to them by her behaviour. Two factors are of importance here. First, the group was classically avoiding a situation that could reveal its 'bad' feelings by directing attention onto someone who openly broadcast her 'badness'. Secondly, because of Elisabeth's appalling home conditions, accepting the role of scapegoat fulfilled her deep need for attention and status. As we shall see in Chapter 10, this kind of dual fulfilment of needs poses extra problems when any attempt is made to resolve the whole process.

Michael

In this case Michael was a member of a mixed youth club in the age range 15–17. His peers found him masturbating in the toilet. The factors of situation and character which promoted his victimisation were as follows:

- Michael – a quiet, retiring, colourless member of the group – a follower.
- Response to situation by peers – disturbed, disgusted and given to ridicule him.
- Group – church-based and activity-oriented with very strong leanings towards doing the 'right' thing.
- Outcome – Michael was scorned, teased and made a common butt of obscene jokes.

- Group motivation – masturbation was currently an area of fantasy and guilt among the group as a whole.

Heap emphasises that the promotion of Michael as the group scapegoat was accidental in that had he not been discovered in the toilet he would not automatically have become the group victim. Other differences can be noted to the case of Elisabeth, in particular that no need of Michael's was met by the scapegoating process. The sole gainers in this case were the group members, who were able to transfer their own guilt and fears about masturbation onto Michael. In this case there were no real indications of a potential scapegoat, only a situation that was loaded with emotional potential. Indeed, any member of the group by similar action could have become the group's victim. As lasting damage could result from such an attack, this situation required and received urgent management attention which involved the overt support of the victim and an attempt to bring all the other factors to the group's notice to be dealt with.

Anne

Anne was a member of a leisure-time club for young patients in a psychiatric hospital. At the time of the victimisation the club was producing a play, and the factors that placed her in the role of scapegoat were as follows:

- Group activity – the whole process of putting on the play was going wrong.
- Anne – appeared to function at about the same level as everyone else in the group. But she was convinced that she was worthless and had attempted suicide. She was manipulative in that she used situations and relationships to affirm her own lack of worth. She was suspected of having considerable feelings of hate towards her parents, which she controlled by directing them against herself.
- Group response – the members blamed Anne for everything. She could neither learn her part nor be relied upon; she was stupid and crazy.
- Group need – was to be able to blame someone for its own shortcomings and its own organisational inadequacies and to lay off the possibility of being compelled to recognise these deficiencies by blaming them all on Anne.

In these circumstances the scapegoating fed two sets of needs as had the same process for Elisabeth. In Anne's situation, she had drawn all the blame onto herself not by directly offering herself as a victim or by provocative behaviour, but because her peers had sensed her need to affirm her own worthlessness and were quite relieved to put onto her their own feelings of not being able to cope, which was being clearly demonstrated all around.

The situation was dealt with by the group leader by ensuring that the drama production was successful. While recognising Anne's particular problem, the group leader also realised that the scapegoating related specifically to the drama production situation, and when this was satisfactorily dealt with the actual need of the group to blame someone for failure would disappear.

John

This is something of a special case as John was accused of leading four other boys of previously good character into a programme of malicious damage and car stealing. The main points about John and the situation are as follows:

- Personality – physically weak, relatively unintelligent and possessed of few social skills.
- Background – parents divorced, he lived in an otherwise all-female household in poor housing in an area of noted criminality. He had been in trouble on several previous occasions.
- Other group members – came from respectable backgrounds, were intelligent and obedient boys – they had not previously associated with John – were conforming youths with no previous hints of rebellion but appeared to have been frustrated by all-encompassing parental control.
- Needs – John needed to be given attention; the group members needed to be shown how to give expression to their aggression and their urge to rebel.

As Heap suggests, John's previous record made authority assume that he was the one who dragged the others into criminal activities. But a closer look at the logisitics would indicate that this was far too facile an assumption. The needs of the 'good' boys to express aggression towards their parents was blocked by fear of the parents' power and they then set up a situation where, by appealing to the vanity of someone with experience, albeit less intelligent, they pushed him into a leadership role and were thus able to lay all the blame for their actions onto him, and very convincingly, when they were caught.

Conclusion

All four of these episodes indicate that the differences which make a group choose one of its members to bear the blame for the group's behaviour or feelings are very wide ranging. Indeed, the common factor in choice of victim can be seen to be that the scapegoat in each event did something or was something that actually fitted the needs of the group at that moment. This leads me to suggest that, aside from deliberate provocation, the choice of victim may rest not nearly as much upon a particular array of characteristics or behaviour as upon an essential and powerful need of other group members to purge themselves of very specific bad feelings.

Of all the victims discussed above, Anne is probably the only one who would be scapegoated in many situations because it was not simple attention she required but confirmation of something that she already implicitly believed about herself and would presumably have sought in any company – that is, her own worthlessness.

We must conclude then that coincidence of need and attribute combined are far more likely to produce the process of scapegoating than either alone.

When scapegoat victims are considered in some detail a certain complexity of evidence arises which tends to obscure a clear analysis. Put simply, this involves being able to decide whether the symptoms and behaviour exhibited by the victim *pre-dated* the initial acts of scapegoating, and could therefore be considered to be instrumental in the choice of that particular person as a victim, or whether they arose as a *direct result* of the conflicts and distress caused by being made a victim.

Bell and Vogel (1970:386) repeatedly assert that in the families in their survey the children who were victimised *became* subject to severe tensions and their behaviour deteriorated. Indeed, they argue that one of the most important factors of selection was an apparent instinctive realisation on the part of the scapegoaters that, because becoming a victim so incapacitated a person, the chosen victim had to be someone whose contribution to the family unit was small and/or one that could be taken over by another family member.

But then we are faced with ample evidence that victims become scapegoats because they are different in some essentially notable way, or, and this is but one particular but very powerful kind of difference, their behaviour portrays a large irritant quality which is ultimately provocative and, even at the best of times, tends to elicit tart responses. It is precisely this distinction between pre-victimisation provocation and difference and post-victimisation behaviour patterns that causes problems in the analysis of the process and of the kind of people who become scapegoats. For however an individual is selected to fulfil the scapegoat role, if that individual does not escape from it in some relatively short time then there will be an obvious escalation of those character-istics of that person which caused him or her to be selected in the first place. Indubitably, if provocation and an irritant quality were not major sources of choice as a victim, then what deterio-rates or escalates about the victim's personality and behaviour must be those attributes which most concern the scapegoaters. Put in simple terms, the victim develops and displays precisely those characteristics of which the scapegoaters wish to rid them-selves.

Part III

Theories and explanations

In the preceding chapters I have tried to show how the scapegoating process was relevant to those societies in which it was practised. Indeed, how it arose as a result of, or rather as part of, a belief system that was based upon the fear of punishment for wrong-doing by supervisory and all-seeing gods.

The fact that as societies became larger and more diverse and eventually increasingly secularised no corresponding decrease in scapegoating activity took place – in fact, quite the reverse – can only lead to speculation that scapegoating in some form or other meets a basic human need to avoid censorship and blame. What has changed as society has changed is not that need, but essentially the focus of the propitiatory act. In most lives gods apparently no longer occupy a supervisory and regulatory position, which is now, to all appearances, taken by the society itself or at least by some particular and all-important part of that society. There is some evidence that not all perceptions of divine supervision have disappeared even among those sections of society who would categorically deny any religious belief, but it has assumed the status of a superstition or a vague acceptance of factors like fate and luck.

In fact, scapegoating has become very much a pattern of social behaviour and has, as we have seen in the examples offered earlier, been accompanied by a huge increase in rational intent. No longer can we accept that scapegoating is a ritual or even a symbolic act, for in a large number of instances it is clearly being employed as an objective strategy designed specifically not just to ensure survival in the face of hostile censure, but actually to maintain the status quo. The cost of error is thus borne by others, and so the element of sacrifice still exists.

Of course, as we shall see in the theories and explanations that follow, this rational strategic approach is not always the case. Many scapegoating activities appear to arise from the need to discharge tensions generated by both known and unknown factors in social situations and the whole process becomes one that may operate well below the level of the conscious understanding of its perpetrators and masked by them with what appears to be extremely logical rationalisations.

None of the explanations that follow, either of the process or of the victims, is entirely satisfactory. Those which offer motivations operating below the level of conscious understanding, omit the fundamental analysis of why human beings cannot confront and accept blame for their behaviour. Why has the twentieth century developed so many theories and approaches to the development of human beings which all have as their basis the need to accept responsibility for our own actions and to cease the undignified and selfish attempts to shuffle off blame onto others, if this were not some basic element of human behaviour? Those ideas which stress that scapegoating is the result of the conscious use of a deflective strategy omit to discuss why such a transfer should be deemed to be a possibility. All say little or nothing about the all-seeing, all-knowing entity which motivates individuals and groups to attempt to evade blame in the first place, especially if we know that it is in some degree, if not entirely, justifed.

Self-justification – the need to be right, to feel that we are good, to accept that the benign images we have of ourselves are true – may be essential to our confidence and to our continued existence. Why then do we develop therapies and encounters which attempt in secure surroundings to challenge, to confront and to adjust those self-images to what are decreed by the practitioners of such approaches as more authentic or more valid, and so on?

One thing is certain: the attempts by human beings to transfer blame for their own actions, to accuse innocents of responsibility for disasters and to attempt to propitiate and deflect the forces of criticism have in no way abated over the totality of humanity's existence and must therefore be accepted as an essential ingredient of social behaviour.

Chapter 7

Attempts at understanding: the process

In modern times the term *scapegoat* has been used to describe a relatively powerless innocent who is made to take the blame for something that is not his fault. Unfortunately he is not allowed to escape into the wilderness but is usually subjected to cruelty or even death.

(Aronson 1980: 212)

Because scapegoating has become a phenomenon of social behaviour and ostensibly the mystical and ritual factors have disappeared, the process has been subjected, like most other aspects of human behaviour, to the scrutiny of social scientists, journalists and other curious and sometimes involved people in attempts to understand what happens. The problem, as with all aspects of human behaviour, is that what is apparent and observable and often in appearance simple, can stem from the most complex and bizarre motivation. Indeed the difference between the perceptions of individuals crucially involved in an incident and those of non-involved observers marks one of the problems quite clearly.

Jones and Nisbett (1971) showed that whereas those involved in a situation believed that their actions were a direct response to their perception of the nature of that situation, observers of those actions believed that they were basically derived from the personality of the actor. Thus an individual A would say that he responded with anger to a situation in which he found himself because the situation caused him to feel anger. Whereas observer B would be more likely to adduce that A's anger stemmed from the fact that A was a choleric individual.

Another problem of understanding behaviour lies in the apparently irresistible drive to discover causes, which of course leads into theorising about them on the basis of the evidence of behaviour and consequence. But as we shall see, and indeed have already noted, neither behaviours nor consequences that are observable can be wholly depended upon, let alone causes which inevitably are infinitely more concealed.

The theories and explanations presented here are as diverse as they are interesting, but they serve to add considerably to our understanding. Because causes are almost always inevitably hidden, what we are presented with are ideas which fit the observable facts with some degree of elegance and with marked economy.

Scapegoating seems to have both rational and deliberate sources as well as irrational and hidden ones. For instance, the examples given earlier include illustrations where individuals and groups, finding themselves the centre of some difficulty and being held responsible for some minor or major catastrophe, deliberately and consciously set about deflecting the blame, laying the censure and hostility onto some other selected individual or group. Self-preservation may well be the basic motivation for this kind of manoeuvre, plus a somewhat cynical disregard for the welfare of others, but the essential point is that it is a rationally conceived if exploitative gambit.

The irrational form of scapegoating seems to occur when the basic energy required to bring about change stems from frustration, usually of the normal response to a particular stimulus. The major factor here may well be that the level of consciousness about the frustration and the frustrator can be quite high, but the understanding of the need to discharge such an uncomfortable level of distress may be less so and the method of so doing seemingly dependent upon opportunity. There are many sayings throughout the world which have as their basis the blind rage which strikes at innocents who have had no part in its production.

Human nature being what it is, there are most likely elements of both rational deliberate intent and apparently irrational behaviour in the process of scapegoating. But whatever the constituent elements may be, scapegoating is largely a group phenomenon. But in a small group or large organisation, when individuals or groups are scapegoated, the process is dependent upon the majority belonging to the group of those who scapegoat, and a much smaller number, often a solitary individual, who become the victims. The proposals of one of the major theories, that of displacement, tend to illustrate the thesis by showing the displacement of frustrated anger of an individual onto a victim, but the process is equally possible within a small group or an organisation.

> The literature of the social sciences and related professions reveals two basic perspectives on such processes. Scapegoating, for example, has been posited on the one hand to be a resultant of group efforts to foster or maintain integration, and on the other to be primarily a consequence of the specific provocations, deviant behaviors, or ineptness of scapegoated individuals.
>
> (Feldman 1969: 30)

Feldman's dichotomy may be too simple but it serves to highlight the two perspectives that will be pursued here. In this chapter we shall look at the process from the point of view of those people who are or who become scapegoaters and, as we shall see, there are many more possible explanations of the practice than that of fostering or maintaining group integration or even of responding to provocation. Indeed, scapegoaters do not have uniform motivations, but we can draw a clear distinction between those whose behaviour is apparently irrational if not entirely random and those whose behaviour is decidedly rational from their point of view and produced with the obvious intent of deflecting from themselves opprobrium and blame.

IDEAS AND EXPLANATIONS – 1

There is also the difference between the original position of having being put under tension by others and events, and the methods adopted for relieving oneself of it. If there is no felt or perceived pressure, there is no scapegoating. So our first task is to discover what actually generates the energy, the discharge of which can emerge in the form of scapegoating. In terms of the explanations available it is necessary to look at ideas of:

- Frustration, aggression and displacement
- Projection and psychic discomfort
- General hostility

- The personal characteristics of scapegoaters – the authoritarian personality.

Frustration, aggression and displacement

Scapegoating, or picking on an innocent person, is a familiar example of displacement in the face of threat.

(Medcof and Roth 1979: 206)

In 1939 Dollard and his colleagues published their findings on the frustration/aggression hypothesis (Figures 7.1 and 7.2), and this thesis has been the guide for a great deal of the research into aggression ever since.

In its simplest form the hypothesis states that frustration produces a readiness to aggress, and that aggression is always produced by frustration. Frustration is defined as the blocking of a sequence of goal directed acts, and aggression as a response with the goal of injuring an organism or object.

(Geen 1972: 2)

Simple and direct as this thesis is, it has been challenged in many ways. For instance, aggression does not simply arise from frustration. Individuals may become aggressive in order to attain desired ends. Sometimes people are stimulated to perform acts of aggression by exhortation or, as witness Milgram's (1974) experiments on obedience, as an ordinary response to authority. Then there are the effects of stress, of crowding and of the possibility that human beings are instinctively aggressive and that this basic nature erupts when social control diminishes. It has also been mooted that aggression may be genetically determined.

Another difficulty with the frustration – aggression hypothesis is exactly how far is frustration responsible? It is generally recognised that frustration

may not have simple effects on aggressive behaviour but may represent one element in a complex set of cognitions that interact to determine behavioral outcomes.

(Geen 1972: 2)

Thus there are suggestions that frustration must contain a large element of perceived arbitrariness and injustice for it to precipitate aggressive acts. Indeed, there is evidence pertinent to scape-

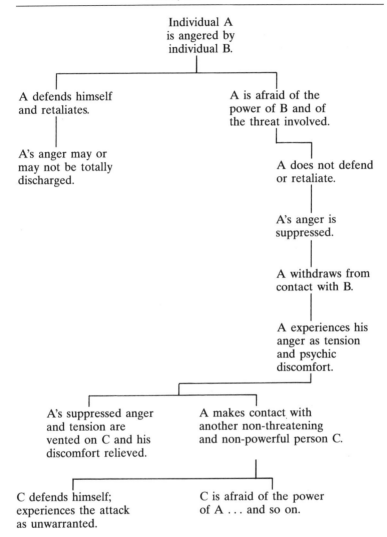

Individual A
is angered by
individual B.

A defends himself
and retaliates.

A's anger may or
may not be totally
discharged.

A is afraid of the
power of B and of
the threat involved.

A does not defend
or retaliate.

A's anger is
suppressed.

A withdraws from
contact with B.

A experiences his
anger as tension
and psychic
discomfort.

A's suppressed anger
and tension are
vented on C and his
discomfort relieved.

A makes contact with
another non-threatening
and non-powerful person C.

C defends himself;
experiences the attack
as unwarranted.

C is afraid of the power
of A ... and so on.

Figure 7.1 Frustration, aggression and displacement: chain of events
on a one-to-one basis.

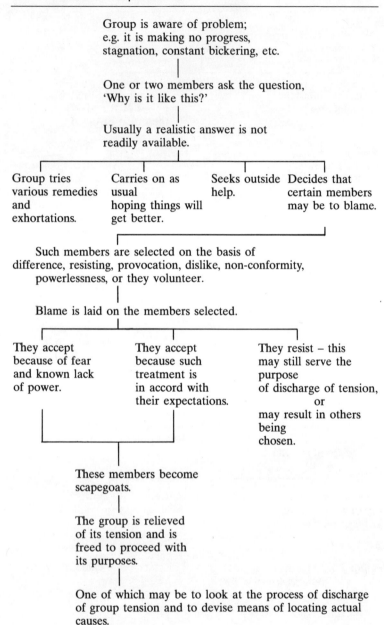

Figure 7.2 Frustration, aggression and displacement: chain of events
in a group.

goating which suggests that where frustration is seen as accidental, or resulting from sources well beyond the control of the frustrating individual, the resulting hostility tends to be displaced to some substitute. Thus it would appear that scapegoats may be used as a method of release from frustration when the frustrated perceive that the problem arises from circumstances which occur without malicious intent and over which there is apparently no form of control.

Another element to consider is that frustration often tends to produce a form of inertia based on the fact that there appears to be no way to resolve the difficulty. Aggression demands action and can thus free the frustrated from this sense of helplessness and can endow the aggressor with some sense of purpose and achievement in the form of discharge of tension.

MacLennan and Felsenfeld (1968: 28) write:

> conditions for scapegoating include a high level of tension (anger, anxiety, guilt, frustration); a person or section of the group against whom the members could rightly feel angry but for one reason or another are not able to express it, and a group or member who is seen as different, vulnerable and open to attack.

It is appropriate that the authors lump all the main drive factors together under the rubric of 'tension', for the simple reason that the experience of tension in a group or organisation is a much more common experience than that of the composing drives. From the point of view of being able to recognise the energy source of the scapegoating procedure this is a valuable point, as we shall see later.

Finally there is some need to consider that aggression as a response to frustration may be imitative in that there is evidence that aggressive behaviour tends to increase or intensify when examples of aggressive behaviour in others are plentifully available.

Projection and psychic discomfort

Projection is an unconscious mechanism in which certain feelings or intentions – in general 'subjective' states – are erroneously attributed; the true location of the feelings is in the person projecting, not in the person or group to whom the feelings are attributed. Thus when guilt is the 'frustration', the feelings or intentions that occasion the guilt are first projected upon another person or group, then that other person or group is made a scapegoat.

(Johnson 1961: 595)

Johnson goes on to add that projection and displacement are primarily defence mechanisms which help to relieve the tensions of psychic discomfort. Tension is an uncomfortable experience and sets up a degree of dissonance, but also generates an energy potential which, until it is discharged in some way, continues to irritate.

Drever (1952) suggested that projection emerged as an interpretation of people and situations in which our own experiences and feelings were attributed to those people and situations. He also suggested that these feelings were almost always unpleasant ones such as guilt or of inferiority and the whole purpose of projecting them was to justify ourselves in our own eyes.

Hinksman (1988) offered three reasons for projection, which were that there were aspects of ourselves which we found to be socially inconvenient or because of seeing ourselves as being socially respectable bound by introjected rules which we see being broken by others and by establishing possible comparisons with others by fantasising being that person.

Ryecroft (1972) wrote that projection was preceded by a denial, 'one denies that one feels such and such an emotion, has such and such a wish but asserts that someone else does'.

In order to feel comfortable with ourselves we apparently need both to be able to justify our feelings and actions and to be able to displace those we do not find acceptable onto others.

Similarly the process of scapegoating, when the group blames a member for particular ills and tries to get rid of that person, suggests that some hated aspects were present in other group members and being avoided. Parataxic distortions, the individual's proclivity to distort his perception of others also provide valuable material which go to make up the work of the group.

(Aveline and Dryden 1988: 51)

What is relevant here to the process of scapegoating relates to the discovery of unacceptable parts of the self, the projection of them onto others and ultimately the banishment and punishment of those others for possessing those unacceptable traits, behaviours and intents. If one adds to this some of the factors of cognitive dissonance (Aronson 1980) – which would imply that if, when needing to feel good, the individual discovers that he or she possesses 'bad parts' – a dissonance of that individual's perception of self is established which is distressing, and by far the simplest method of discharging that distress is to punish others for having the same kind of 'bad parts'. Thus, the act of scapegoating, i.e. transfer of blame or of badness, takes place.

What is true of individuals is equally true of groups and organisations. They, too, can split the complexity of human experience into either good or bad parts, can feel the same distress at seeing that they are hosts to both and can endeavour to discharge the bad by transferring it to others by a process of believing these others to be possessors of the 'bad parts'.

Like all the other explanations as to how scapegoating seems to occur, this one also pays little attention to how victims are chosen. But it does hint that the choice might partly depend upon the chosen actually possessing some, in however small a part, of the 'bad parts' which are to be projected in much greater quantity.

Perhaps the most important aspect of this form of explanation of the scapegoating process is the fact that it points up what would seem to be an innate need of human beings to discharge the tensions engendered by the development of a recognition of the possession of unacceptable attributes. If what is revealed about human need in this way by modern forms of investigation into behaviour is supposedly devoid of any belief in mystical or religious causation, then there is a strong case for suggesting that the ancients also possessed this need in equal measure. Thus the factor which shaped their response to the need was the belief system in which they lived. This, in turn, has something to say about the belief system, if such a unitary entity can be said to exist, of today's scapegoaters. At first glance this would seem to imply that a modern belief system would be constructed round the primacy of self-preservation in much the same way as was that of the ancients. However, the threat that was being defended against is no longer the punishment of a god but of a society and, indeed, what may be only a selected part of a society. We shall need to explore this aspect of scapegoating in more detail later because, although projection may be an unconscious defence mechanism, there is a great deal of evidence that the process of modern scapegoating derives a considerable proportion of its momentum from conscious and deliberate attempts to evade responsibility and blame on the part of the scapegoaters by a process of deflecting and diverting attention onto others.

General hostility

> The scapegoat has always had the mysterious power of unleashing man's ferocious pleasure in torturing, corrupting and befouling.
>
> (François Mauriac 1961)

There is some evidence that human beings possess a generalised hostility to those not of their immediate community. Storr (1968), discussing intolerance and the paradox of scapegoated minorities who are made victims because they are in a weak position but can still be regarded as potentially powerful and thus dangerous, suggests that because we are able to identify with another person and imagine what life may be like from his or her point of view, we can also have some idea of that person's suffering. But Storr says that from this identification can come both compassion and cruelty. He indicates that our own dependence and helplessness as babies creates the possibility of identifying with the humiliated: 'Scapegoats personify both power and weakness at the same time. We project the former attribute upon them and identify with the latter characteristic' (p. 98).

Taken at its simplest level, this statement could be intended to imply that ordinary people have hidden paranoid tendencies to believe logically untenable facts about others. In addition, it also suggests a proclivity for brutality in identifying with and taking pleasure in making others suffer.

While somewhat startling as a basis for scapegoating activity, there has surely been sufficient evidence in this century alone of the paranoia of people and of the almost unbelievable brutality that human beings can inflict upon one another. Given the right circumstances, particularly where survival is, or apparently is, at stake, we are all capable of considerable acts of humiliation and brutality. Logically it would not be necessary to preach the effi-cacy of loving one's neighbour if hostility and suspicion of others were not a common human experience.

Most of the ideas that surround suspicion and hostility are related in some way to ignorance, prejudice and, inevitably, the perception of difference. They are also related to personal esti-mates of value which result in some people feeling, often for no good reason, superior to others. As a spring, a source of energy, hostility, envy and difference are extremely powerful. Such a cocktail when it exists in a social situation can produce a society which is extremely dissatisfied with its position and in classic frustrated form unable, as far as it is aware, to do much about it. Thus it requires but an incident to act as a trigger and the latent hostility can produce an eruption in which others will suffer by being blamed for the situation, and most likely punished for it as well.

It has been suggested that the basis for suspicion and hostility may well stem from from harsh and threatening parental disci-pline which develops in the child a high degree of insecurity and hostility towards the parents.

> This combination sets the stage for the emergence of an adult with a high degree of anger, which, because of fear and insecur-ity, takes the form of displaced aggression against powerless groups, while the individual maintains an outward respect for authority.
>
> (Aronson 1980: 214)

The personal characteristics of scapegoaters – the authoritarian personality

> lack of insight into one's own shortcomings and the projection of one's own weaknesses and faults onto others is often found in high scoring subjects (high on the authoritarian attitude scales). It probably represents the essential aspect of the mech-anism of scapegoating.
>
> (Adorno *et al.* 1950: 233)

As we have just noted, general hostility and suspicion may be the source of energy which can produce the scapegoating pro-cedure. What Adorno and his colleagues sought to demonstrate was that there are individuals who are predisposed to be prejudiced. As Aronson writes: 'not solely because of immediate external influences, but because of the kind of people they are'. Such people tend to show certain characteristics, viz.:

* Their beliefs are held with great rigidity and inflexibility.
* Their value system is ordinary and conventional.
* They cannot tolerate what they describe as 'weakness' either in themselves or in others.
* They believe that people should be punished for transgression of the conventional social code and that we should make no attempt to understand them.
* They show a high level of suspicion, particularly with regard to the unfamiliar.
* Constituted authority is regarded with an enormous degree of respect and entails a high degree of obedience to its order.

It can be seen that individuals with such marked characteristics are susceptible to frustration to a great extent and are unable to tolerate it. Nor can they tolerate the idea of being responsible for the frustration, and are thus extremely likely to lay the blame for misfortune and impediment upon others. The self-righteous and self-justifying nature of the authoritarian personality would lead to any tolerance of blame being highly unlikely. It would hardly be regarded as a possibility to be considered, and thus the source of frustration *has* to lie elsewhere. Given this state of affairs it would seem inevitable that not only would the onus tend to be directed towards those who did not possess the same rigid beliefs, and were regarded as weak, but that they would also be visited with punishment.

If Adorno is right, then it must be accepted that a particular form of human personality can fulfil most of the basic and necessary criteria for initiating the process of scapegoating – almost, it would seem, without the need of a situational trigger.

IDEAS AND EXPLANATIONS – 2

In the following sections, ideas and explanations which are directed at conscious avoidance techniques and about the factors that influence the way scapegoaters choose their victims, are offered for consideration. Some of these ideas have mirror images which emerge when we consider the role of the scapegoat. For instance, deviancy is a perception of difference and non-conformity from the viewpoint of the scapegoaters and others, but it may equally well be seen to be a deliberate and conscious choice of behaviour pattern by the person who becomes a victim.

- Conscious avoidance and victim choice
- Deflection – a rational defensive measure
- Protection of self-esteem
- Attribution theory
- The dislike hypothesis
- Propinquity, availability and restricted choice
- Situational factors.

Conscious avoidance and victim choice

What has been described as the strategy of maintenance in modern group systems is essentially a survival technique, and in this sense bears a direct resemblance to those ancient techniques discussed earlier. There are, of course, differences. Most of the survival techniques of the ancients were related to the cycle of crop growth and seasonal changes in their available food supply. Thus their rituals tended to be annual in the sense of preparing for a new season. Modern maintenance techniques are not so essential to actual total survival as those of old but tend to relate only to a situation which is only a part of each participant's life. Also, they are not based upon any actual perceptible cycle unless this is fixed in a system by the nature of its structure or imposed on it by the larger structure in which it is embedded. Modern maintenance strategies tend to be applied at the point of observable breakdown or, probably more accurately, at the point where breakdown, total or partial, is observed to be imminent. They are, as the name implies, strategies for keeping the system running, and while there are some elements which are applied on a routine basis in the same way that mechanical, electrical and other systems are maintained, the more important strategies are applied to what might be termed 'unexpected deteriorations'.

There is, however, a great deal of difference between a maintenance technique that is essentially a repair job, and thus positive, and one that saves the organisation by a process of victimising one or more of its members. As we have seen, scape-

goats really are victims in the sense that their hurt and humiliation is deliberately engineered by others in order to deflect
censure from themselves. But there are also scapegoats whose
role is classical in the sense that they are being sacrificed in order
to preserve the group or organisation of which they are a part.
Having placed all the bad feeling that was impeding the progress
of the group onto the shoulders of one selected victim, the group
members are psychologically free to pursue their goals with
renewed energy, relieved of the drag of problems.

This basic assumption of relief brought about by the maintenance gambit is one that we must consider very carefully as it is
often offered as a reason for tolerating scapegoating.

Johnson (1961) describes the role of scapegoat as 'integrative
and tension-managing'. Thus by implication he is suggesting that
the process has a sustaining and positive effect. Essentially this
thesis is prepared to accept the victimisation of some of its members as a valid cost of maintaining a group or organisation as a
functioning entity. It is, however, a cost that those members may
not be so willing to pay. But if the process of scapegoating does
actually manage to keep the group in existence *and* the situation
of the salvage operation is analysed to try to understand why it
worked, then without doubt the events can possess meaning
beyond the actual process and may serve to highlight what needs
to be done with the next crisis when it arises.

Considered in this way, the maintenance gambit is a stop-gap,
an emergency ploy activated to meet a situation in which either
the time to devise other techniques to meet the situation or the
knowledge, or both, is not available.

Storr (1968) believes that pariahs 'serve a valuable function in
human communities for the discharge of aggressive tension'. In
this sense scapegoats tend to be pariahs. The valuable service
they offer is to free communities from debilitating tensions, which
is achieved by the scapegoats becoming the focus of the discharge
of aggression. The justice of such behaviour remains questionable
except in terms of the greatest good for the greatest number.
However, the basis of scapegoating, being a maintenance operation, is founded on that conception and thus the victimisation
of some is a cost which the community as a whole is prepared to
pay.

Hinshelwood (1979: 218), in a book titled *Therapeutic Communities*, wrote: 'the emotional life of a community consists to a

large extent of a wide ranging exchange system for unpleasant emotions'. Later he added that a therapeutic community 'usually contains special individuals who act as a kind of a *sump* into which negativity and bad feelings tend to drain, and who become scapegoats or prophets of doom'.

The value of maintenance techniques is that the group or community survives, but unless, as noted earlier, the group then uses at least some of the time gained by the manoeuvre to consider not only the costs but also the causes and methods of coping in the future, then the 'some must die that others may live' syndrome will be repeated as being the most effective gambit on offer, no matter what it costs the victims. Maintenance in this case then sets off a system in which it becomes more important to find a suitable victim than to discover the actual causes of difficulty.

To continue the 'sump' analogy, it might be worth while taking a passing glance at the concept of deviancy.

Dentler and Erikson (1970) put forward several propositions about the function of deviancy in groups which, if we are prepared to accept that scapegoats are group deviants, may be worth considering. Their propositions covered the following behaviour:

• 'Groups tend to induce, sustain, and permit deviant behaviour.'
• 'Deviant behaviour functions in enduring groups to help maintain group equilibrium.'
• 'Groups will resist any trend towards alienation of a member whose behaviour is deviant.'

Dentler and Erikson are stating that deviants have a maintenance function in a group; indeed, they go so far as to equate deviants with high status leaders as being on the margins of the group and as possessing specialised status. Like leaders, deviants are regarded as giving the group structure or 'shape' in that the deviant is a focus, an individual about whom the group constantly reminds itself that some action should be taken and because of whom the group is more certain of what it stands for and what it can or cannot do.

By defining such an individual as deviant, Dentler and Erikson are placing stress upon personality and how this affects the structure of the group. There is no clear proposal about how the defined behaviour arises although they say that 'deviant behaviour is a reflection not only of the personality of the actor, but of the structure of the group in which the behaviour was enacted'. Yet, in Proposition 1 they assert that deviant behaviour can be 'induced' by the group, presumably in order to acquire the beneficial effects such a role enforcement can produce.

There is no great difference between enforcing a deviant role upon a member as a group maintenance ploy and the scapegoating processes we are investigating. In both instances the processes of selection need careful analysis to discover the reasons for choosing a group member to be either a scapegoat or the occupant of a deviant role. In both cases the costs to the victim may well be little regarded in the light of any equilibrium and maintenance gains to the group.

Deflection

> The motif of the *malefactor scapegoat* does not derive from the belief that evil is something concrete and indestructible, but from the belief (or theory as we might prefer to call it today) that evil is a quality of intended behaviour.
>
> (Kraupl-Taylor 1964: 14)

In his relatively idiosyncratic approach to scapegoating, Kraupl-Taylor postulates two kinds of scapegoats: the one that purifies and the one that is a malefactor. The former is synonymous with the classic ancient ritual form but the latter is interestingly different.

Here the basic motif is one of punishment, which has itself two forms. To quote the author (p.15):

> Their punishment (*the scapegoats*) can be regarded as a safety device that propitiously deflects the same fate from us for the sins we have ourselves committed. Alternatively their punishment can be viewed as a preventive device that obviates further malefaction by either the original culprit or others.

The first form of punishment is concerned with the universal desire to escape from the consequences of our own wrong-doing. Thus certain individuals have always been encouraged to perform wrongful acts openly during a prescribed period of time, at the end of which they have been punished usually with death – a fate they were willing to accept in return for a period of licence, e.g. Saturnalia. When the punishment was complete the rest of the involved society felt that the dead person had suffered punishment for them all and they had assuaged their guilt vicariously.

The second form of punishment is visited on wrong-doers who are significantly different from the rest of us and whose punishment makes us feel superior because of the apparent enormity of their behaviour.

In both instances Kraupl-Taylor has suggested that the main objective of the procedure is the survival of the complacent and self-satisfied majority, but it is interesting that he feels it necessary to classify those who are sacrificed to this survival as malefactors, in effect as wrong-doers. Doing the wrong thing is only one manifestation of the general concept of difference, which is the usual basis for the selection of a scapegoat. Indeed, being too good is sometimes an equal basis for being selected. The general underlying motif is that of highly noticeable difference which, when coupled with dislike and a perception of an inability to protect themselves, forms the criteria of selection of a victim.

Protection of self-esteem

> While self-preservation occurs in all cultures, it is of greater importance in some. In most of the East there is great anxiety about losing 'face', so that self-preservation is of great importance.
>
> (Argyle 1976: 87)

What passes for the appearance of public figures is more often than not a very consciously controlled projection of an agreed image. But because reputations are based upon such publicly presented persona, those who have them and who support them have a vested interest in maintaining them.

> When an individual appears before others, he knowingly and unwittingly projects a definition of the situation, of which a conception of himself is an important part. When an event occurs which is expressively incompatible with this fostered impression, significant consequences are simultaneously felt in three levels of social reality, each of which involves a different point of reference and a different order of fact.
>
> (Goffman 1969: 234–4)

The three levels of social reality referred to here were social interaction, the individual personality and the society. Goffman infers that such an incompatible event produces consquences in all three areas, viz.: the interaction between the public figure and the 'audience' is disrupted because perceptions have changed and positions that were firmly held previously are no longer tenable. As Goffman puts it, 'the minute system created and sustained by orderly social interaction becomes disorganised'.

This disruption brings about a considerable drop in the perceived reputation of the individual as a competent performer, which then tends to diffuse to his organisation, his supporters and others close to him. Finally, incompatible events, disruptions of the image presentation can have a devastating effect in discrediting the individual in his own eyes.

Given that Goffman postulated such consequences for public figures when disruption of an image-presentation occurs, it is somewhat strange that he did not even hint at the ways in which so valuable an asset, both to the individual and his organisation, could be protected. However, Argyle (1976: 387) provides us with several protective devices which may be employed in the face of serious challenge to a person's self-image. They are briefly:

- Selective interaction: the individual moves away from those people who are setting in motion the challenge, towards those who have a more congruent view of the challenged person.
- Changing standards of comparison: the challenged person moves away from challengers towards people whose standards are more in keeping with his or her own.
- Conformity to group norms: the challenged person deliberately produces behaviour and appearance that is more in line with the accepted norms of the challengers.
- Reduction of value allotted to the opinions of the challengers: the challenged person chooses to disregard the opinions of the challengers as worthless.
- Disbelief: the challenged person disbelieves or ignores evidence that any challenge is being made.

However, the first two of these protective gambits involve a movement away from the challenged person's public or group, and such a move is often neither possible nor to be contemplated because survival within the group is the whole reason of the challenged person's existence and no alternative position exists.

The others depend to a great extent on the kind of behaviour or appearance being challenged and the other sources of power possessed by the challenged person. The remaining method of protection is to provide a focus for the challengers which is not the individual originally selected. This is the way of the scapegoat or the substitute.

Substitutes can be bought both by payments of value or by appeals to honour and the good of the organisation. Alternatively they can be thrust into the substitute position because they have no option, being unable to defend themselves by reason of power-lessness, threat or even by being a willing sacrifice for their own personal ends. Substitutes are frequently persuaded to protect others on the grounds that those protected are of inestimable value to the cause, whatever that might be, e.g. in terms of the work they alone can do. But in most cases substitutes are, in, all senses of the words, scapegoats or fall guys.

Fritz Heider (1958: 14–15) said that scapegoating behaviour: 'Often is not simply release of aggression, but includes blaming others for changes which, if attributed to the person, would lower self-esteem.' Heider believed that scapegoating exonerated indi-viduals from any blame for their own condition. He also hinted that this behaviour was conscious because he uses the terms 'excuse', defined as denying the attribution of a bad act to oneself, and 'imputation', the act of ascribing bad acts to others. The idea of imputation concerns Heider quite considerably, and he quotes evidence of it as a pathological state in the form of imaginary accusations, noting that the psycho-analytic interpretation infers that such imputation is used to bring an end to painful internal conflicts, usually of sentiments condemned by the individual's conscience. The mechanism, of course, is still one of projection.

However, excuse and imputation are also to be found on both sides of the rational/irrational divide. As our earlier examples have shown, the process of blame-laying and the evasion of responsibility, powered by a purely selfish urge to survive, can and does take the form both of excuse making and, more impor-tantly for our purpose, the imputation of fault and indiscretion, etc., onto others in the hope, frequently justified, that this manoeuvre will deflect the attack onto the chosen focus.

Attribution theory

> To ask people to refrain from assigning blame, responsibility or
> credit for events until 'all the facts are in' is to ask them to do
> a very difficult thing. Our cognitive organising processes force
> us to jump to conclusions about causes.
>
> (Raven and Rubin 1976: 77)

Attribution theory assumes that we have almost a compulsive
need to ascribe causes to observed behaviour, as the quotation
above suggests 'to jump to conclusions'. The basic assumptions
of the theory are that human beings are equipped with dispositions, e.g. to be kind, to be generous, lazy, etc., and that from
these dispositions arise intentions which, modified by personal
knowledge and ability, are applied to social situations in the form
of actions. But all we ever see are these actions and thus the
whole basis of their pre-existing structures back to the dispositions can only be inferred.

The theory is very general and applies to all forms of human
behaviour but in the case of scapegoating it seems to plot a clear
inferential path from the awareness of difficulty and frustration
back through the behaviour of certain members of a group or
organisation, to their intentions and, eventually, to their dispositions. If the ultimate conclusions reached on this backward trip
are that the intentions were negative and unhelpful and that the
dispositions were unconcerned or hostile, then the powerful need
to blame someone for what is occurring can find a readily acceptable focus.

Attribution theory can offer an explanation of the way in which
the need to blame actually is laid at the door of a particular
person or group and it does have the added bonus that it includes
the concept that behaviour provides the stimulus for the backward search and ultimate blame.

Raven and Rubin (1976: 79ff) offer, as an example of the
operation of attribution, the trial of Lieutenant William Calley
who, in 1970, was held to be responsible for the massacre of a
whole village of unarmed Vietnamese civilians and convicted of
war crimes. In a survey in 1972, Kelman and Lawrence discovered
that those who disagreed with the court's verdict gave two main
reasons for considering the decision unfair. The second was: 'The
trial used Lt. Calley as a scapegoat: one young lieutenant
shouldn't be blamed for the failures of his superiors.'

The arguments for and against are both versions of attribution theory. Those who thought Calley was guilty assumed that he was morally responsible for his actions. They reasoned that he must have had both the understanding and the ability to have a choice of options. Thus because he ordered the killing he must have wanted this to happen – in effect he was a criminal.

Those who argued against the court decision saw him not as a criminal making a deliberately evil choice but as a victim – he did what he did not because he wanted to do it but because he was doing what he had been ordered to do and he was responding to the situation as he found it. His knowledge and ability would not have allowed him to do otherwise.

Significantly, as Jones and Nisbett (1971) point out, the reaction of actor and observer involved in an incident tend to be disparate and thus it is that in a blame-laying sequence the scapegoaters who play the role of observers tend to see the behaviour of the victim as being solely related to his or her dispositions and intents, and as they are perceived to be negative the victim is therefore blameworthy. The victim, on the other hand, may well quite truthfully say that his or her actions were a response to the situation as seen. The outcome tends to depend on two major factors: the first is the degree of urgency necessary to relieve the frustration or to sort out the difficulty in which the group finds itself; the second is the degree of difference and dislike that is accorded to the victim and his or her behaviour by the majority of the group or organisation.

This process is reasonably clear in that we do ascribe actions to the personality and characteristics of the actors almost as if it was not possible to observe behaviour without attributing some cause to it. If other pressures are great enough, then those attributions will tend to be very purposeful but even less accurately based upon verifiable evidence than usual. Thus the concept of innocent victim is realised.

Dislike hypothesis

Putting it simply, the present argument holds that the aggressive tendencies engendered by frustrations are generalised to those groups whose perceived characteristics result in their being disliked.

(Berkowitz and Green 1965: 34)

This is one of the possible explanations of scapegoating which applies almost as equally to the victim of the process as to the perpetrators. Berkowitz and Green argue that given qualities of victims, in this case the victims of prejudice, act as a stimulus which triggers the hostile and blame-laying activities. They also argue that the characteristics which seem to be the most important are those which incite intense dislike.

It must be reasonably obvious that dislike can be engendered by a great many behavioural acts as well as personal characteristics or even beliefs. The major factors which incite dislike may well be based upon a simple perceived difference; however, Berkowitz and Green state that strangeness and difference are potentially the stimuli which incite hostility when danger or apparent threat is also present. Now this looks somewhat like a circular argument until it is made clear by the authors that the dislike, which is the factor that draws the frustrated anger of scapegoaters, actually pre-exists that frustration.

Therefore, while people may be tolerated in a society even though their behaviour and personal characteristics are significantly different and thus somewhat threatening, they do not necessarily become scapegoats until and unless the society becomes frustrated by its inability to cope with some major crisis – that is, until the level of aggression becomes intolerable and has to be discharged. Then those who were disliked but tolerated become the victims of that aggression and are usually blamed for the crisis.

As Berkowitz and Green say: if negative attitudes exist towards a particular group in society, it does not matter how these attitudes arose, what is important is that as long as they exist the group on which they are focused is 'a likely target for displaced aggression'. If the reasons for the general dislike of a particular group have some bearing or relationship in kind with society's frustration, then the probability of displacement of aggression becomes very much more likely.

Availability, proximity, propinquity

Aggressive responses to frustration that cannot be expressed owing to inability to attack the actual frustrator are stored up until a weaker, less powerful target for aggression is found as the scapegoat. But who picks the scapegoat? Why is the target invariably designated by the most powerful in society – are they the most frustrated?

(Carolyn C. Sherif 1976: 116)

Carolyn Sherif neatly highlights the distinction between the arousal of frustration, the need for it to be suppressed and the choice of target for its eventual release. Most of the explanations and theories of scapegoating we have looked at so far have been concerned with the origins or nature of the frustrations that provide the essential drive for scapegoating. But it must be obvious that the process of scapegoating, whether it is a discharge of pent-up frustration or the deliberate deflection of hostility, requires a target or targets.

To begin at the simple end of this problem we need look no further for a beginning answer than to the idea of propinquity or availability. Most persons or groups who are scapegoated are not only already known to the scapegoaters, they are also usually reasonably physically close to them in the same organisation or group. The reasons are fairly obvious. In the process of laying blame, or of finding a victim on whom pent up anger and frustration can be released, several factors are of great importance.

As the frustration was caused in the first place by the differential in apparent power between the frustrator and the frustrated, then the latter has to be reasonably certain that any target he or she may choose has to be less powerful than the selector. He or she cannot know this unless the target is reasonably close and well known. The element of powerlessness must be well authenticated or the whole process of frustration may be repeated if the target can retaliate or defend. Equally, if the process is a conscious one of deflection of blame, then the scapegoater has to have reasonable certainty that the displacement target is one who will be liable to be accepted as such and, moreover, is one who has little chance of evading, deflecting or resisting becoming a victim.

All these requirements can usually only be met when the scapegoaters discover that they have adequate knowledge about the proposed victim. Of course their assumption of adequate knowledge may be wrong, but it stands less chance of being so if the victim is not only in close proximity to the scapegoaters but also known to them.

Furthermore, the choice, as we shall see, is often based upon the characteristics and behaviour of the proposed victim, knowledge that is usually only available to those in fairly constant contact with one another. It is not feasible, for instance, that a victim could be targeted on the basis of his or her provocative behaviour, or perceived difference or on resistance or lack of conformity, all of which form the main stimuli for scapegoating if both victim and scapegoaters did not occupy contiguous space for long periods of time.

There are exceptional circumstances where a stranger or strangers may enter a group or a community and be recognised immediately as potential targets for aggression. The criterion of availability is fulfilled here, but the knowledge of potential has to be based upon an instantaneous perception rather than upon knowledge gained from long contact. The reputation that precedes such people is often the culprit. But it is recognised that some people seem to be scapegoated wherever they go, and it must be inferred that there is something about their appearance or behaviour which provokes an almost immediate recognition that they are potential victims. This may have something to do with the fact they appear to have an expectation of being victimised and that in a resigned way they accept this role as part of their costs of existing.

Situational factors

Instead of leading towards self-confrontation, tribal myths point outwards, towards self-glorification and self-aggrandisement. Such myths derive their impetus and energy from insecurity, from blindness, from prejudice and from the wilful creation of a scapegoat.

(Baigent et al. 1986: 159)

The anthropological view of past behaviour expressed here is still common enough, and politicians use it very explicitly. By fostering a myth about an external group it becomes possible to displace the energy surrounding domestic difficulties and failures and focus them onto the out-group who then are seen as adversaries and scapegoats.

Outside groups, on the other hand, also lend themselves as a projection screen for wishes and fears, often so strongly repressed in the high scorer (*authoritarian attitude scale*).

Immoral tendencies are easier perceived in, or ascribed to, groups which seem not fully assimilated or altogether foreign. Hostility and the fear of being victimised can be expressed against these groups without restraint or expectation of retaliation. Even if such out-groups as the Jews are described as powerful, it is the knowledge of their ultimate weakness which makes them suited for scapegoats.

(Adorno *et al.* 1950:485)

Cultural factors are factors of extremely visible difference. But, as Adorno and his colleagues pointed out, those differences are significant only insofar as they catch the attention of people whose personality would rate a high score on the authoritarian attitude scales. The burden to be discharged cannot be off-loaded willy nilly anywhere, and suitable targets needs must have the necessary qualifications, i.e. they are believed to be weak, immoral, different in so many dislikable ways and incapable of retaliation.

Johnson (1961) maintained that although the choice of scapegoat may seem to be irrational, it is never random, there being at least a symbolic connection between the victim and the frustration of the scapegoaters. He says: 'Although the victim is "innocent" his place in the social structure does have something to do with his being victimised' (p.597).

MacLennan and Felsenfeld (1968:87) suggest that scapegoating may be used as a testing device in groups. They believe that the process works by a member of the group being deliberately scapegoated in order to find out what reaction this will provoke in the group leader. Thus they can find out whether the group leader is safe and can be trusted and also what kind of care the leader takes of group members. The authors also record the use of scapegoating to promote 'collaborative resistance' – that is, when most of the members of the group are engaged in the activity of scapegoating it tends to bind them together. Such bonds as are established may then be sustained in other areas of group activity by becoming the basis of a mutual support system.

In the groups of adolescents which MacLennan and Felsenfeld were discussing, it is interesting to note that what they call 'the most usual form of scapegoating' involved the transfer of anger away from the leader to a member of the group. However, there is little evidence in the literature on scapegoating of the process

being used as a definite technique to engineer given consequences, although there are other references to testing out processes.

SUMMARY

What seems to emerge with some clarity in this brief survey of
the suggested explanations of why individuals and groups become
involved in the scapegoating process is the simple dichotomy
between those explanations implying conscious intent and those
indicating unconscious impulse.

In this context it is interesting to note that while there is
nothing difficult to understand about the survival element of
consciously applied strategies like the deflection of accusation
and speculation from one person to another, there are some
problems about those elements which have been defined as
unconscious. In effect, a considerable number of the explanations
in this category have a simple form which comprises the assumption of a large element of stored energy generated by unexpressed
anger, frustration, personality characteristics, etc., which are then
discharged by the operation of a situational trigger. The release
of energy and emotion always has the characteristic of being
inappropriate to the situation that fired it. That is, it is largely if
not entirely unexpected, it is probably infinitely more powerful
than the situation would logically demand, and it contains large
punitive and sacrificial elements.

It can thus be agreed that when scapegoating possesses what I
have called 'inappropriate' elements to a marked degree, then
any method of dealing with the process must take into serious
consideration that what is being produced is a process that is not
understood by the scapegoaters and will therefore be defended
and explained by rationalisations.

Finally, it must be remembered that what have been presented
here are explanations – that is, attempts to understand a complex
social event – which fit the observable details but do not possess
the quality of first-order facts with sustainable proofs. The basic
use for such explanations is to present a coherent basis for understanding and, if required, for any process of intervention that
may be necessary to alleviate, mitigate or avoid harm.

Chapter 8

Attempts at understanding: the victim

What makes an individual or a group become the victims in the scapegoating process?

> Blaming the victim is a common reaction to crime among police, politicians and ordinary citizens alike. If your house is burgled, you should have installed burglar alarms. If your car is broken into, you shouldn't have parked it where you did. If a young woman is raped, she shouldn't have been wearing a short skirt, or walking home by herself.
>
> (Mary Kenny 1993)

Given the fact that such a tendency exists, and that it is a kind of scapegoating in itself, it is necessary to be extremely careful in presenting ideas and explanations of the scapegoat role. Considerable attention has been paid to the fact that scapegoats may well excite others to the point of promoting their own victimisation. Any consideration of the victim role in scapegoating has therefore to examine why particular individuals appear to be chosen for victimisation and others do not. There have to be reasons, and any review of the literature will immediately suffice to show that it is almost universally believed that there are certain defining characteristics and behaviours of those individuals who become scapegoats.

Now this is very close to saying that scapegoats become scapegoats because they deserve to become scapegoats, which is in fact blaming the victim for being a victim. Crude though this statement may be, it contains an element of truth because, as we shall see, one of the major factors that appears to focus attention on a potential victim is 'difference'.

By itself, this is a wholly inadequate explanatory device. Indeed, difference of its members is often the most productive asset that a group or organisation may have. So a difference which focuses the attention of the scapegoaters has to be a difference which is provocative, disliked, inept or possesses some characteristic that is not only different but engenders hostility and aggression.

There are also many substantial explanations of scapegoating that indicate that the victim chooses the role rather than attracts victimisation without intent to do so. Once again there is a great need for caution. Without doubt, there are individuals whose isolation and lack of positive relationships makes any relationship – even a humiliating and hostile one – preferable to no relationship at all.

We can start our study of explanations of the process of becoming a scapegoat by looking at ideas related to the personal characteristics and behaviour of victims, their lack of social power, their stimulus qualities and their differences.

> Jake was singled out by his rather shapeless figure and rubbery face. He served as a scapegoat wherever he went, and clearly provoked his peers into bullying him.
>
> (Button 1974:23)

From the outset it must be made clear that in any examination of those individuals and groups who are scapegoated by others, the role of victim has a certain complexity which defies a simple analysis based upon obvious factors like difference and deviance. Thus it is helpful in the early stages of examination to define four categories of victim, viz.:

1. Scapegoats who can be described as volunteers.
2. Scapegoats who are definitely selected by their scapegoaters.
3. Scapegoats whose occupancy of the role is permanent, probably in any group of which they are members (like Jake in the quotation given above), but certainly in some groups.
4. Scapegoats whose occupancy of the role is transient, dependent on the existence of a particular situation within the group, e.g. resisting change and development when everyone else has accepted it.

As with all classifications of complex social behaviour these categories are too simple. Indeed, in many scapegoating situations a combination of these factors is probably at work to produce the end result. For example, a scapegoat may be deliberately chosen by his or her group peers but the reasons for the choice may lie as much in the chosen one's apparent willingness to accept the role as any other criterion of choice. Again, situations may develop in a group or organisation which actually throw individuals into the public arena; they are neither volunteers nor deliberately selected, but they are obvious choices to have heaped upon them the bad feelings of their colleagues. Such scapegoating behaviour may be transient and fade when the situation that brought it into existence changes, but it may also mark the scapegoat as a person who can be cast in that role on other occasions, whatever the situation.

Of the four categories listed above, the difference between those scapegoats who are regarded as temporary and those seen as permanent may be of prime importance. Indeed, the form of scapegoat referred to as 'permanent' is also often called 'classical' or 'traditional' and is characterised by the victim possessing all the intrapsychic factors readily recognised as those associated with the traditional scapegoat, with all the psychological mechanisms of becoming a scapegoat and of the scapegoating process in place.

On the other hand, the temporary scapegoat tends to arise because he or she is seen as different in some way, but often that individual is in some way resisting or handicapping the group's progress to at least some of its goals. In this case, because the group's new position requires to be consolidated and may be fragile, any resistance or hindrance is usually met with anger and frustration which, as we have seen, are some of the bases of the process of scapegoating. Such resistance also serves to remind the group of the closeness of possible failure. Depending upon the stage of development reached by the group, the effect of seeing a member displaying frustrating difference may be great or small, but by being related to a particular circumstance is usually transient and, indeed, has a maintenance quality in that it can act as a catalyst to the group and spur it to make further developmental efforts.

SOCIAL POWERLESSNESS

And finally, the data also revealed that scapegoated members were characterised by significantly lower social power — the likelihood of exerting social influence — than their peers.

(Feldman and Wodarski 1975: 92)

As part of the theories of displaced aggression, scapegoats are traditionally described as those seen possessing very little social power. Indeed, when we want to look at the ways in which intervention may be made into the process of scapegoating, we shall see that Feldman (1969) recommends that one indirect method is to attempt to increase the perception of others involved of the actual worth of the scapegoat. If perception of the value to the group – that is, possessing attributes which will materially assist a group in the pursuance of its goals – is generated, this immediately confers upon the individual so perceived what French and Raven (1959) described as specialist power.

The main areas in which individuals chosen as victims lack social power are as follows:

- weak enough not to retaliate
- extremely low in influence
- directive, high participator attracting blame through lack of sensitivity
- ineptness in group tasks
- no control over incidents of aggression
- isolated
- low status – 'untouchable'.

The original thesis of powerlessness is quite firmly based in common sense. Few people will target their frustration and aggression on individuals whom they consider will be able to defend themselves or to retaliate with the possibility of inflicting hurt. Indeed, as we have seen earlier, the whole foundation of the frustration/aggression explanation is that of displacement away from some source of frustration which is regarded as too powerful for successful retaliation onto others. These, by virtue of being chosen, are seen as being in the same position *vis-à-vis* the scapegoater as he or she is *vis-à-vis* the original source of frustration – that is, powerless.

However, in this respect there are several points to consider. First, there is evidence that those selected as scapegoats are not always powerless; in fact, they may sometimes be exactly those seen to be very powerful – for instance, when a group puts its leader into the scapegoat role. The reason adduced for this phenomenon is that the group feels that the powerful person has led the group into difficulties and should have known better and, even more important, should be able to get them out.

Second, because of the common marked inefficiency of the assessment of personal characteristics, the person selected to be scapegoat may be chosen on the basis of a very poor assessment of capability. Many silent and uncommunicative group members have been set up for the scapegoat role, and the scapegoaters have discovered that silence was not an indication of weakness but a measure of independence and sometimes of considerable personal strength.

Berkowitz and Green (1965) criticised the so-called 'safety' hypothesis in the selection of victims and suggested that when strong members of a group were chosen as scapegoats the process was concerned with what the authors called 'status recovery'. This process works on the basis that frustration generates hostility only when it is successful in lowering self-esteem. By not attacking weak members of the group but some of the most powerful, group members can relieve their frustration by blaming someone for the misfortunes of the group and at the same time bolster their own self-esteem in that they were strong enough to tackle fairly formidable members of their own group.

There is some overlap with characteristics which indicate low social power within the group and those which engender the dislike that seems to be a potent selective factor in scapegoating. Thus, where members are seen to be resisting group progress or performing group functions with a huge degree of ineptness, it may be difficult to assess whether these factors are precipitated by low social power or whether they are just personal characteristics of the individuals concerned. When groups are struggling against odds to execute their function and achieve their goals, such individuals often add to the frustrations that other group members feel, and in some cases the members are quite justified in doing so.

Many of those selected to become scapegoats are members who have moved or been forced to the edges of the group. They are isolates of low status whose opinions are of little concern, and indeed are seldom heard because they have no skills to gain a hearing and are seldom if ever offered an opening by others. They may, in the past, have been aggressive in an uncontrolled way, letting the group down and been rewarded with the role of 'untouchable', their presence in the group tolerated but not valued except as those who act as the sump for all the bad feelings in the group. Their presence *is* tolerated because the group knows that if they were to be rejected then other members of the group would have to take on the role of scapegoat as and when the need arose.

DISLIKE

Once again, the factors that have been noted in the literature to generate dislike in peers overlap, to some extent, with the personal characteristics of chosen scapegoats. This is inevitable and results from looking at the same social behaviour from two different angles, one being the characteristics of the actor and the other the responses of observers of those characteristics.

> Putting it simply, the present argument holds that the aggressive tendencies engendered by frustrations are generalized to those groups whose perceived characteristics result in their being disliked.
>
> (Berkowitz and Green 1965: 34)

Berkowitz and Green were referring to groups that were scapegoated, but the reference applies equally well to individuals within groups. The major characteristics listed in the literature which promote dislike in peers are as follows:

- similarity to the frustrator
- perceptibly different from others
- deliberately provocative
- low commitment to group norms
- low liking for peers
- displays attention-seeking behaviour
- resists group progress
- complains about being abused or exploited
- operates as spokesperson for the distressed
- private attitudes and public statements are discrepant
- expresses dissatisfaction with the group and position within it.

As can readily be seen, all the factors in this list are obvious sources of irritation, especially to group members who are already somewhat harassed by circumstances. Indeed, some of the characteristics listed here are the exact opposites of those that are usually quoted as forming the basis for friendship or attractiveness in others. For example, in *Groups* (Douglas 1983: 100–1) I quoted Nicholson's (1977) six factors in the formation of friendship:

- The need for stimulation or arousal.
- Reassurance: the need for confirmation of values, attitudes, and to gain support for the image we have of ourselves.
- Similarity: we tend to like people who are like us.
- Recognition that friendships are expendable.
- Proximity: we tend to like people whom we meet regularly (in essence this contains the idea of availability) and we cannot really like people whom we never have any opportunity to meet.
- Physical attractiveness: usually stronger earlier in our lives before we begin to use non-physical assets as the basis of our assessment of others.

It is interesting to note that 'proximity' promotes either liking or disliking, according to other factors in the equation. Thus, because the potential scapegoat is close enough to be seen frequently, all the irritant characteristics are clearly visible. Added to the factors which cause either personal like or dislike are those which denigrate the group and its purposes, obfuscate its goals and handicap progress. When these are allied to complaints about ill-treatment by the group, and other obvious differences, then it is quite clear that such group members who are kept there on sufferance for reasons best known to the group are the obvious ones to be sacrificed on behalf of the group's welfare.

PERSONAL CHARACTERISTICS

> ... the object serving as the target for the intolerant person's aggression usually has certain stimulus qualities for this person, and that objects not possessing these characteristics are less likely to be attacked.
>
> (Berkowitz and Green 1965: 31)

The problem of highlighting the personal characteristics that prompt a group to select one of its members for the scapegoat role is very familiar. The literature records lists of the characteristics that scapegoated individuals have been seen to possess. It may be true to infer that these characteristics caused their possessors to be selected in the first place, but that cannot really be substantiated unless there is considerable evidence to show that people possessing these characteristics, and being members of groups, are the primary targets of scapegoating in all circumstances. To my knowledge this evidence does not exist. But from the amount of data collected about those who are victimised in this way – and given the theoretical assumptions that victims are usually those who are regarded as weak or who have irritated the group in some way or who are disliked or different – it is reasonable to record the list of salient characteristics.

For instance, MacLennan and Felsenfeld (1968: 28) gave the following list of characteristics and behaviours which they had discovered were displayed by potential scapegoats. They

- possessed provocativeness, high anxiety, irritating mannerisms or superiority, and seemed to imply that they knew more than others;
- appeared more virtuous;
- possessed more and flaunted their good fortune;
- had different interests from the rest of the group;
- did not accept the values of the group;
- were the sickest or the weakest.

These authors were writing about groups of adolescents, but when comparing their list with those recorded by others about groups of adults the similarities are quite marked. For instance, Garland and Kolodny (1966: 204–6) compiled the lists presented below.

Those factors within the individual which tend to precipitate scapegoating:

- Inability to deal with aggression from others.
- Strong passive or masochistic mode.
- Inability to cope with own angry feelings.
- Tendency to be burdened with guilt.
- Has a need to seek rejection, ridicule and punishment.
- Has a confused sexual identity.
- Produces attention-seeking behaviour.
- Appears to have a poorly organised or insufficient aggressive drive.
- Is perceptibly different in some obvious way.
- Expresses a marked ambivalence to the most cherished persons in the group.

To this fairly extensive list may be added the further characteristics of:

- Shows no evidence of adaptive learning.
- Lacks perception of the fact of being persecuted.
- Displays deviant behaviour.

The list becomes quite formidable in presenting traits that are
exactly those calculated to irritate and provoke group members,
especially when they are already in some form of difficulty.

Garland and Kolodny's definitive paper on scapegoats suggests
other ideas. For example, such individuals repeatedly put themselves in contact with people and situations which, on past experience, have proved to be injurious and harmful. This characteristic
is based upon past performance and seems to show either a
marked inability to learn from past experience or that such harmful situations are actively sought. Thus, when such situations actually arise it would appear that the scapegoat actively seeks to
intensify them and to push potentially dangerous situations into
fruition.

This leads to a series of events which can be shown to follow
the pattern of provocation after an attack, which draws forth
retaliation and protestation that, having been attacked, the victim
is only acting in self-defence. If this protestation is questioned
then the victim consistently denies that there is any pattern of
persecution or that he or she is actively seeking it. Occasionally
the response seems to vary to some recognition of what is happening, but with a strong statement that bad as it may be it is
beyond his or her control. It is just 'one of those things'.

Any examination of the list of characteristics credited to potential scapegoats would seem to indicate that virtually anything can
focus the efforts of scapegoaters in given group situations. But
the factors they all appear to have in common are that whatever the chosen characteristics may be, they all are indicative of
marked differences between the victim and his or her persecutors
and that perhaps as a result of these differences, but perhaps also
for other reasons, the potential victim is often intensely disliked.
Indeed, it has been recorded that some scapegoaters have suggested that there were ethical reasons for selecting and attacking
a particular individual. In other words, they felt they were morally
justified in so doing.

Mann (1967) put forward an interesting thesis of the 'sexual' scapegoat. Thus, along with other roles that group members play, such as 'moralist', Mann defines the role of the 'sexual scapegoat' as deviant and suggests that it is 'most commonly observed'. The description of this role seems to imply that the individual seems to be 'particularly immature or inhibited in some aspect of the sexual domain'. Mann gives examples of the mockery and derision that this entails. The description bears some resemblance to the 'confused sexual identity' put forward by Garland and Kolodny.

Mann estimates that two factors are involved in this situation:

1. The attack on the scapegoat may be the usual displacement by some members of their feelings towards the leader.
2. The group deflects its anger from what they fear – that is, the leader's condescension and ridicule – onto the non-retaliatory victim.

Mann believes that all resisters are scapegoated, particularly if at the time the group has just made some progress which is still relatively fragile. He says that the sexual scapegoat is most often a male member who appears to his peers to be very uncertain of his own masculinity and attempts through confession or other ploys to offer himself to the group as a case well worth study. These individuals are characterised by being unremarkable and assume 'a dependent, loyal and somewhat distant stance to the leader. They are consistently low on enactment . . .'. As the group develops, these individuals become increasingly dissatisfied with the group and their own place in it; they become increasingly hostile and disturbed and begin to complain that they are being exploited or abused in some way. Mann suggests that these feelings tend to emerge with most force when the group is going through its internalisation phase.

On the sexual scapegoat, Mann (1976: 237) states:

> In most respects he is no different from many other minor members. There is, on the other hand, one distinctive preoccupation which seems to precede his ultimate deviance. The sexual scapegoat is likely to express an extraordinarily intense ambivalence to the Hero. He is impressed by and attracted to the Hero, but finds him too frightening and primitive to be tolerated. He often seeks the companionship of the most distressed and withdrawn females in the group, occasionally

appearing as their spokesman, most often presenting himself as a fellow sufferer. He oscillates between attempting to dominate and speak for the distressed females and describing himself as even more forlorn and put upon than they.

As the group improves its capacity to develop, it needs to distance itself from those members who display dependence, inhibitions and incompetence which derogate the group's increasing but fragile independence, potency and competence.

Mann's thesis lends itself to the idea that the behaviour which attracts scapegoating comes into play when the group has reached a certain stage of development. The groups he had studied were set up to learn about group development and were, to that extent, somewhat more self-regarding than other groups. But the idea that individuals are scapegoated when the group reaches a stage of development in which certain members cannot contribute is widely documented elsewhere. If this analysis is taken further it would imply that each stage of development in a group would tend to produce the need for a scapegoat unless it was an easy transition from the previous stage. Mann's thesis, although superficially describing the kind of person who is scapegoated, is most basically concerned to present scapegoating as a maintenance technique that is employed to protect the group at those stages of transition when its development is at its most vulnerable. It also implies that the group is aware that the next stage of development may be more difficult and that progress towards it cannot take place while there are some members who have still not fully absorbed the current change.

DIFFERENCE

The scapegoat may be selected in the first place on the elemental basis of being different. He may be isolated because of difference of age, sex, religion, class, race, etc.

(Foulkes and Anthony 1957: 205)

Foulkes and Anthony list here some of the principal differences which they refer to as 'elemental'. They are not only extremely visible differences but also possess a strong factor of irritation to others. Difference, in this essentially negative aspect of its role in groups, is surrounded by ignorance, prejudice and a strong element of fear. Quite simply, differences that are accepted when all is going well, and may even be seen as helpful, can quickly become the focus of fear, dislike, prejudice and ultimately of victimisation.

Most of what has been stated about scapegoats has involved the concept of difference, and there is little to add here except to look at the different types of difference and make some indication of what potentiates them and draws the distinction between those differences that form one of the group's basic resources and those that serve to mark out individuals for a form of victimisation.

> There are thus two kinds of DIFFERENCE involved, and the distinction between them is essential. Analog differences are differences of magnitude, frequency, distribution, pattern organisation and the like. Digital differences are those such as can be coded into DISTINCTIONS and OPPOSITIONS, and for this, there must be discrete elements with well-defined boundaries.
>
> (Wilden 1980: 169)

Most of the differences which seem to precipitate scapegoating behaviour in groups and organisations would appear to be differences of magnitude. Scapegoats seem to be picked on the basis that they have either more of some characteristic or less of it than the majority of their peers. In normal circumstances a great deal of this difference would be used by the group as resource material in order to broaden the range of members' understanding. Thus difference of itself is seldom the basis for scapegoating; it has to be accompanied by the strangeness that is provoked by what Feldman (1969) called 'intense personal dislike'. As we have noted earlier, difference even accompanied by dislike can be tolerated in a group until that difference comes to be regarded as deleterious to either the continued existence of the group or its progress in achieving its aims, or to represent aspects of other members about which they are ashamed or guilty.

> The deadly combination of low commitment to group norms, inadequate performance of important group functions, low liking for peers, and low social power practically ensures scapegoat status for a group member.
>
> (Feldman and Wodarski 1975: 93)

One final point about differences needs to be made. It is the primary fact of difference itself – visible, clearly distinguishable difference which forms the focus for the activities of scapegoaters and not, in the first instance, the nature of that difference. Of course, as Feldman and Wodarski point out, if any particular difference is also accompanied by other factors, such as low commitment to group tasks, incompetent performance, etc., then as a focus of scapegoating attraction the difference becomes so much more certain to be the focus of victimisation.

The use of such differences to form the basis of scapegoating is highly unethical and is essentially a form of oppression. In our multi-cultural society the problem of racial discrimination makes the issue of racial difference very sensitive. Such a difference possesses many of the essentials that can make it a victim-focus, and much attention has been given to this fact.

I would like to stress that while such victimisation is deplorable in the extreme, there is a clear need to demonstrate the process exactly for what it is, i.e. survival at the expense of others. It is also necessary to point out that, because it is an important and current social issue, an overemphasis on racial difference as a victim-focus can obscure the development of a truer understanding of victimisation in general.

In a single gender group, or in a single race group, scapegoating will take place. When people are desperate, and particularly when no apparently reasonable explanations of the cause of that desperation are available, then even the colour of one's hair may well be sufficient to attract the opprobrium and blame that the group needs to discharge. It is the measure of the intensity of the need to survive that prompts apparently civilised human beings to behave with such an element of injustice to their colleagues.

Prejudice must also be considered because this can add considerable weight and importance to any factor of visible difference. For instance, racial difference may be an extremely visible difference in a group, and if this is backed by a considerable degree of prejudice – i.e. members having expectations of behaviour and attitudes based largely on a lack of actual knowledge – then the racially different can be an easy target for victimisation. This appears to be so, even when the crucial factor of the visible difference having some degree of similarity to the nature of the group's dilemma is not present.

Thus, it can be said that where scapegoating takes place the first element of choice of victim is the presence of difference. Second, where difference is compounded by other factors such as dislike, inadequate performance, unacceptable behaviour in regard of group norms, then the selection of such a member as a victim is almost assured. The third compounding element occurs when the appearance, behaviour and difference of a member bears some close resemblance to the basic dilemma of the group.

Part IV

Management

Given that scapegoating is a pattern of social behaviour and not a mystical ritual, then it follows that it may be considered to have beneficial and deleterious consequences in certain different circumstances. In the following chapters we are concerned, primarily, with the recognition of the scapegoating process – which is no easy matter for it has to be differentiated from very similar circumstances in which blame is a reality and, even more importantly, where blame is apportioned partially on the basis of reality and partially on victimisation. It will also be necessary to make an analysis of whether what is occurring is a benefit, and for whom, and of how that beneficial form or forms may be used. Finally, we shall consider methods of coping with those forms, which may cause substantial damage either to individuals or groups as the cost of their implementation.

Our society is much given to devising and using ways of changing attitudes, beliefs, behaviours, opinions, etc., of which society – or at least some influential sections of that society – disapprove, or which can be demonstrated to be harmful either to their possessors or others. Thus, although scapegoating may be an extremely efficient manoeuvre in maintaining individuals, groups and organisations intact through periods of difficulty, the cost of success may well be considered to be too high. Indeed, this is often the opinion of scapegoats, except for those particular victims who occupy the role from choice because it supplies certain needs that they cannot achieve elsewhere or in other circumstances.

In Chapter 9 we look closely at what those costs might be, what rewards they ensure, and whether indeed the balance is productive of long-term maintenance or merely of a stop gap or desperation measure. Following on from assessment of the scapegoating situation we shall then discuss how it can be managed to ensure maximum benefit to the group and minimal damage to individuals. The processes of control will usually be operated by a group leader or other with responsibility for the group's well-being and functional efficiency. Consequently, Chapter 10 is concerned with what can be attempted in the way of resolution when the cost/reward analysis is heavily weighted in favour of the former, even when long-term survival is taken into account.

The terms 'management' and 'resolution' are used here in the sense in which they were employed by Frey (1979: 124) in her analysis of the methods of dealing with conflict:

> Management refers to the reduction of tension in the conflict in order to enable the person to pursue his or her goal. Resolution means that the individuals work to reduce the conflict until both parties are satisfied and/or the individual is satisfied in cases of intrapersonal conflict. Not all conflicts can be resolved, but with training, they can all be managed more effectively.

Chapter 11 is an attempt to draw together all the threads that have been exposed in the course of examining the process of scapegoating and the victims of that process. It reaffirms a theme which occurs continuously from the earliest forms of propitiation to the latest forms of the deflection of censure, which is what would appear to be an adjunct to the instinct to survive, and can be described briefly as an unfailing need to evade blame and punishment. The atonement element and the expiatory offer have diminished as part of the blame-laying process; indeed, if there is any large distinction between ancient and modern scapegoating practices it must lie in the drastic reduction of self-blame and of self-sacrifice. If anything, this has powered the scapegoating process with even more force and perhaps with greater injustice than ever before.

Viewed as an element of social behaviour, this factor of injustice is what, by modern standards, requires to be clarified along with the need it attempts to meet, and if possible to be assuaged by approaches that are more just in operation and less harmful. Although the belief system of a modern society is so complex, so diverse and often contains contradictory elements, it is still not possible to explain all forms of the scapegoating process as methods of avoiding the censure of that society, or such parts of it that are significant to the scapegoat. Nor can we complete that explanation by assuming that individual and group needs cover all eventualities. There are still elements of fear of the unknown in our secular and 'scientific' society, elements for which rational explanation does not seem to have any effective or acceptable answers so that there are still beliefs which encompass an all-seeing supervision of everyday activities, all of which add impetus and force to any scapegoating activities.

There is in all probability no satisfactory evidence for this assertion nor any simple answer to the question of what motivates individuals and groups in our society to undertake scapegoating activities, but it is possible to state those questions rather more clearly than heretofore and this is attempted in the final chapter.

Chapter 9

The management of scapegoating

Although many social functioning problems lend themselves readily to analysis and creative action from a traditional group-work perspective, one particularly good illustration is scapegoating behaviour in small groups. The problem is especially germane since scapegoating behaviour clearly involves social interaction between one or more individuals and their peers, has etiological components at both the individual and group level of analysis, and provides useful interventive foci at both levels.

(Feldman and Wodarski 1975: 88)

It was inferred in the introduction to Part IV that 'management' as applied to the problem of scapegoating implied exerting a large element of control to a situation in order to maximise beneficial outcomes for the individual, group or organisation and equally to reduce damaging effects. In other words, it means accepting that a process, in this case that of scapegoating, is in operation and attempting to increase the rewards as against the costs of the process and its aftermath.

It must therefore become apparent immediately that in dealing with what we can call rational/deflective scapegoating, as opposed to irrational/transferring scapegoating, the management problems are significantly different. This, however, only enhances the need for the first and most essential manoeuvre of any interventive or controlling attempt to be concerned to recognise what is actually going on.

While it can be said that the recognition of the process of scapegoating seems to come with comparative ease to observers in society, communities, organisations and groups of all kinds, it must also be said that in certain circumstances major problems with recognition exist.

For instance, in that form of scapegoating in which an individual is being charged with the responsibility for some catastrophe occurring within his or her sphere of operations and, as a result, the individual redirects the blame onto another, there is always the possibility that the person originally blamed may be no more or even less responsible than the individual onto whom the onus was deflected. Because the original blame-laying process was wholly or partly unjust, and thus misdirected, what we see is a process of deflection which markedly resembles the process of scapegoating but which, in this case, is an attempt to secure a more equitable distribution of blame. In other words, in this scenario the apparent scapegoat is actually, or mainly, responsible for what happened. One of the essential criteria often quoted as being definitive in scapegoating procedures – i.e. the innocence of the victim of the responsibility he or she is being compelled to take – is not present. What is being stated here is that because a process of deflection from an accused person to another is clearly visible – particularly in public institutions and large organisations, but less so in small groups – then deflection is of itself a sufficient indication that scapegoating has taken place. The whole process can become very confusing, especially as observers and researchers consistently use the word 'innocent' to describe the scapegoat victim, because it must be obvious to anyone who has had dealings with the processes of survival in public and large institutions, that the 'innocence' of those involved in the apparent scapegoating process may be relative rather than absolute. Thus the difference between the initial accused and the individual onto whom the blame is deflected may well be one of degree – an analog rather than a digital difference.

As I have noted elsewhere, one of the prime factors in recognising the scapegoating process has often been the actual obscurity of the link between individuals and incidents. In most large organisations, responsibility for catastrophe may be extremely difficult to decide for the simple reason that although single, powerful individuals may be seen as the focal point of a decision that seems to have been the root cause of the event, many others will have been responsible both for the process of assessment and for the presentation of information upon which the decision was based, and many more for its implementation in ways that will have been determined by their idiosyncratic understanding of what was required rather than by the original intent of the decision-makers. Of course, those with high responsibility in organisations are traditionally expected, as part of their role, to take responsibility for bad decisions irrespective of the number of others who may have been involved. If this status is sufficiently high, as we shall see later, the preservation of the decision-maker may well form one of the most powerful incentives to find a scapegoat that exist. However, there are still many forms of variable responsibility other than that the focal decision-maker should carry the blame when the whole process goes wrong. It is equally traditional that some of those involved in the process at a different level can be sacrified as scapegoats when it is decided that the focal decision-maker's value to the organisation far exceeds the cost of his or her removal.

In smaller groups there are still to be found high-status members whose influence on decision-making is great and whose value to the group, if only at a particular instant, is high enough for others of lower status to be held responsible for the group's plight as a result of bad decisions. Indeed, resisters – particularly at sensitive times in the group's progress – are often cast in this role and are blamed for the group's difficulties and lack of progress towards its accepted goals. The frustration of group members at this stalled progress makes it relatively difficult for them to assess the actual causes of the stalemate which may well lie in something like their own inability to see the way ahead or in having chosen inappropriate ways of advancing. Thus there is ignorance of the 'real' causes, and so a discomfort and tension tends to dictate that a reason, any reason, must be found. Those who have shown some reluctance to move in accord with the majority of the group's members are thus obvious targets despite the fact that their resistance may have been due to their having a valid perception that the group was going in the wrong direction. They become the focal point of the group's frustration – they are scapegoated.

In this case they are generally accepted as 'innocent' victims. But are they? Not necessarily, must be the answer. It would need some very considerable exploration of what had been involved earlier before it becomes possible to assert that a genuine scape-goating programme had been in operation. Indeed, processes of blame-laying *are* easily recognisable, but recognising the form of that process, the essential step before any decision about consequence or about intervention is made, needs to be more detailed than just a bland recognition that blame is being transferred. There is always the distinct possibility that the action is totally justifiable; and there are always the consequences to be considered, which may actually be benign and rewarding for the group, even if only temporarily, rather than malign and destructive. For this reason we must now look in more detailed form at this process of recognition and search for those clues that might help to decide not just what form of scapegoating is taking place but whether it can, with justification, really be called scapegoating.

RECOGNITION

First, it is necessary to say something about public scapegoating. There are two faces to this phenomenon: that which causes me to call it 'public' scapegoating, and the hidden face which comprises the machinations that are anything but public and take place often within a very small group of people.

The public face of public scapegoating, because it is a matter for the media and for public opinion, does not and cannot concern us here. But the decision-makers whose actions are not public but have consequences that most usually are, can be seen to behave as a small group which will therefore obey much the same rules and follow the same patterns of behaviour as all small groups when faced with a crisis. This being so, no further reference will be made here to the public manifestation of scapegoating, but let it be understood that when either the conscious and deliberate form of transferring or deflecting blame is being considered, the remarks will apply with equal force to the hidden face of public scapegoating.

Having already made some of the salient points about recognition, we can now deal fairly succinctly with the rest. The basis of any successful management of the scapegoating process is founded upon two basic ideas. First, that the form and nature of the process is accurately assessed and, second, that the main thrust of management founded upon this assessment is to maximise benefits from a situation already existing and to limit the possible damage.

The problem of assessing what is actually happening needs very careful consideration, as we have seen, if only to distinguish between blame that is founded in real responsibility and blame that apparently is not. The markers which enable such a distinction to be made are reasonably clear and lie primarily in the group's history.

It must be remembered that scapegoating seldom, if ever, takes place in newly convened groups unless there are very special circumstances, e.g. overt hostility, the need to establish immediately a particular role for a particular person, past experience, etc. It is therefore probable that the type of scapegoating can be based upon a study of the group's history, as it will have been in existence before the process becomes operational.

This past record has several manifest uses but the most important is quite simply that all the past experience of a group will have shown not only a tendency to respond to crisis and problem frustration by the use of a scapegoat but will offer actual examples of such occurrences. This repetitive pattern occurs because the scapegoating process actually worked and maintained the group in existence without a great deal of harm being done, or at least if damage did occur it was considered to be a reasonable cost for what was actually achieved.

The history of a group will also show the roles which various members tend to play, whether as a temporary matter or more permanently. It will also show how members have responded to situations and techniques – both individual and group. There will certainly be evidence of those members who appear to possess the characteristics which, according to cumulative recorded experience, are usually found in those who are most prone to be elected as victim (see Chapter 6). The most obvious of these will probably be the member who is either essentially provocative or apparently willing to become the butt and victim of the group.

If the history of a group can reveal these factors, which might well be called a propensity to scapegoat when pressure, frustration and threat exist, then there is a high probability that what is taking place within a group is scapegoating and not justifiable accusation. Because of the nature of those who are selected as scapegoats, it is usually quite obvious that they are not the sole instigators of the group's problems. As we have seen, they are usually low status and peripheral members, with small apparent capability of retaliating and with often remarkably little influence in the group or in the decision-making process. The probability that they are the actual cause of the group's frustration is therefore low.

However, other group members are also selected to be scapegoats who are not found in the classic pattern just described. They may be leaders or others with power enough to influence group decisions, and then assessment becomes a matter of two prime factors. The first is the actual stage of the group's life at which the apparent scapegoating process is taking place. For instance, many leaders of groups know that at periods of crisis they are blamed by the group for the panic and frustration that ensues. They also know that, although they may be partially responsible, the fact that they are seen by the group as powerful and influential means that the group believes that power should have been used to protect and to guide. Because the group become frustrated, the all-powerful protector is seen to be blameworthy, although the true cause of their tension and discontent may well lie elsewhere – for instance, in their own collective and individual defensive behaviour or in their fear that progress towards their avowed goals is threatening or moving too fast.

Nevertheless, the probability that the selected victim is the prime cause of the group's problem is still a fundamental instrument of assessment.

The second problem involves the resister. Group progress has costs for its members, and each step along the way is often established at a very fragile level. Resisters to any step pose considerable threat to the safety of that fragile gain and can evoke considerable hostility. Assessment here requires that the basis of the resistance needs to be established. Again probability is perhaps the only real instrument available. Resistance to group progress tends to have three main bases. First, the 'resister' is logically convinced that the 'progress' the group is making is either inappropriate or wholly wrong. Second, resistance is based upon an individual's feeling of inadequacy to make the step through fear of consequence, past experience, etc. Finally, there is the deliberate attempt to frustrate and obstruct for personal ends, which is provocative and may stem from a variety of causes varying from downright hostility to the ideas or the persons who support them to an attempt to gain attention.

Individuals do act out of role but they are more consistent in following and producing habitual forms of behaviour. Repetition establishes the way in which individuals function not only in general but more particularly in clearly defined and containing situations such as a group. It may be acceptable to judge that a group member acts in ways that have been established elsewhere and for which he or she may have a reputation, but it is much more acceptable and probably more accurate to assess the probability of a particular role in the scapegoat process being played by an individual based upon his or her performance within that particular group.

When it has been initially assessed that scapegoating is taking place, the next evaluations to be made concern benefit and cost, both to the individuals and to the group. If scapegoating is to succeed as a maintenance ploy, costs must be less than benefits. Essentially the bottom line is that whoever becomes the scapegoat needs to survive as a group member, for if he or she is driven out then the procedure has failed. What then continues to exist is not the group that existed originally. However, where the scapegoat may have been seen to have had some actual responsibility for the group plight, it is not beyond the bounds of probability that the group may have as its scapegoating goal the expulsion of that particular member; e.g. 'If we make it very uncomfortable for him he'll probably get fed up and leave and our problems will be over.' To recapitulate briefly, assessment must include answers to the following:

- Is blame-laying taking place?
- Is it justified – wholly or partially?
- Is it transient or recurrent?
- What are its apparent costs?
- What are its apparent benefits?

Following assessment the group must decide if anything can or should be done about the situation. If the blame-laying is justified then the group has to go through the process of accusation, defence (if any exists) and the consequences of any action they may take – all of which may well be part of the group's normal procedures.

Example

A group that had been set up and funded to deal with finding accommodation for homeless people discovered that their procedures were being constantly undermined by one member who consistently refused to follow the agreed routine.

This behaviour not only frustrated her colleagues but also brought the group into confrontation with other agencies who complained that the group was unreliable and began to refuse to cooperate with any of its members. They, in turn, complained to the unit leader. The culprit defended herself by denying that she operated in an idiosyncratic way and claimed that she was being scapegoated and victimised by the others as a cover-up for their own quite large failures to achieve the group's goals. Because it was a small group the actualities of the so-called victim's behaviour were obfuscated by all manner of personal relationships, rivalries and jealousies. But after a patient sifting of the evidence, enough was discovered to face the member with the fact of her uncooperative behaviour and the group exercised its prerogative under its constitution to ask her to conform or leave. Refusing to accept the evidence of malpractice the member was then asked to leave.

No doubt some of the element of scapegoating actually existed in this case, as witness the various emotional involvements. But there was also clear evidence, from those outside the group, of malpractice and of an almost pathological unreliability plus the fact that the group records showed the essentially provocative and hostile behaviour of the individual in meetings of the group. The cost to the group of maintaining this particular member within the circle would have been to increase their professional isolation to the point where it would have made the unit non-functional.

If an assessment indicates that what is happening in a group is scapegoating, then the steps taken to manage the situation must consider the following:

- Is the process liable to succeed, i.e. maintain the group in existence?
- Is the process well established?

The answer to the first question must be speculative, but if there are signs that the tension which had been present in the group is being discharged then the answer may well be in the affirmative. If the process is well established then the process of management must be the preferred option, bearing in mind that because the process of scapegoating is one of the discharge of tension and bad feelings onto a selected individual, the frustration, anger and fear which impel the action are vital elements in the process of management. Such a strategy of management may be based upon the following lines:

- *Severity of process.* The intensity of the need to scapegoat is an indicator of the amount of energy that may be invested. It is also a fair marker as to whether intervention should (a) go with the process and attempt to maximise its benefits and restrain the damage or (b) attempt to change the whole process.
- *The source.* In many cases the source of the group's tension is hidden from its members and the process of generating insight may be something that is not feasible under the existing state of pressure. It may be a problem of long standing which has never been effectively dealt with in the past, or it may be something entirely new that has precipitated the crisis.

In either case the essential strategies relate to control and guidance of the energies involved, with a degree of protection for the victim.

STRATEGIES

The first and most obvious strategy is to try to talk about what is happening. The limitation on this procedure must be that if management is the principal aim then any discussion must accept the fact that scapegoating is happening and be directed mainly to ensure that this fact is clearly recognised by all concerned. It should also be tempered by the idea that the principal aim must be to gain maximum advantage for the group from the process. Discussion could also include the promise of a review of the process and clarification of the causes, etc., when the existing situation is completed.

Protection for the scapegoat may be necessary, depending upon the situation. Indeed, protection, implying defending, may not be the ideal description of what is actually required and support would cover the facts much better as it contains the idea of protection through enhancing the victim's own behaviour. The fundamental idea is that the process of discharge, which is essential for the restoration of the group's ability to work, shall be allowed to take place or to continue, but that the victim shall be supported by the group leader to:

(a) minimise his or her sense of isolation;
(b) turn aside the more damaging forms of attack;
(c) explain what is happening and indicate what beneficial effect might be available for the group;
(d) insist that the process is a temporary expedient;
(e) promise an investigation into causes, outcomes and alternatives when the group has reached a point of equilibrium.

If the process of attack becomes too intense then more drastic measures for the limitation of damage may need to be taken, bearing in mind that the scapegoating process is already in operation and there may be a fine balance between damage to the group if it is stopped before its cathartic effect is complete and damage to the victim if it continues. This kind of decision cannot be made on any kind of theoretical basis and has to relate to specific and individual situations and assessments.

Progressive reductions in the intensity of the process can be engineered by:

(f) deflection, which amounts to creating a different problem to divert pressure from the scapegoat;
(g) using the power and influence of the group leader role to diminish the intensity of the interaction which may well result in the transfer of group hostility from the scapegoat to the leader;
(h) removing the victim from the group either permanently or temporarily.

In management terms, (f) is a damage limitation exercise and often fails if the intensity of the group's tension is very great. Even if it succeeds it tends to leave a large area of unfinished business so that the main claims for its use are protective plus a perception that the diversion may be a step towards not just management of the situation but to a resolution of it.

In essence, the above three strategies ((f), (g) and (h)) are pro-victim and serve mainly to block the scapegoating process. Because the essential aim of managing a process is to control it rather than eliminate it, their use is basically an admission that control is no longer feasible since the consequences of continuing are too hurtful.

As may be gathered from the foregoing, managing the process of scapegoating tends to be a survival procedure and one which almost invariably is brought into existence when the process of scapegoating is well advanced, is intense and has to a large extent become urgent very suddenly. Basically, scapegoating is a process of unjustified victimisation and although it may indeed maintain a group in existence and carry it through to a period of equilibrium, it is essentially an unethical process. The main value of management is to handle a crisis situation through to calmer waters when the process of discussion, evaluation and hopefully resolution can occur.

Research into group behaviour tends to show that a form of scapegoating occurs in many types of group, where the purpose of the group includes as a main objective some form of development and that the vulnerable states occur as a group moves from one level of proficiency to another or from one stage of a complex task to a more difficult or advanced stage. The change from stable state through a transitional stage to another stable equilibrium is, as we have seen, one that is fraught with dangers, uncertainties and fears of regression.

Scapegoating that occurs during this kind of transitional period tends to be based in fears (a) of being held back and (b) of not being able to cope with the new stage. What then develops is a tension and a need to discharge it. Scapegoats in this situation are often group members who are seen as resisters or mockers, sometimes even those who have made the change from one state to another without apparent effort. The differences from the point of view of anyone attempting to manage this particular form of scapegoating process lie in two fairly obvious points. First, if the process is successful, i.e. the group more or less as a whole achieves the move forward in its progression, then the scapegoating is transient and relatively easily forgotten. Second, the individuals who are usually the victims in this process are not commonly those who would be expected to be selected for that role. The group seems to recognise that this is not so much a discharge of bad feeling or of frustration as that the process of transition is an interval in the development and that the outcome should, on the whole, be a good one. However there is also the fear of failure and if it should occur then scapegoating will almost certainly arise and in a much more virulent and vindictive form than the irritant nature of that which was part of the limbo of transition.

Management here is significant in achieving success. If a group leader is sufficiently aware of the changing state of the group, then an expectation that transient scapegoating will develop almost as a factor of change, will be in place. The essential purpose will then be to highlight the likely transient nature of what is happening and to stress the beneficial nature of the usual outcome.

Example

A group of seven mature and experienced entrants to a social work course met twice a week for an hour and a half for the purpose of learning about group dynamics by the simple expedient of being guided by their group leader, a senior tutor, to examine the processes of their own group. In the initial briefing they had been informed that the contract they should make should be wholly concerned with learning about group processes and that should they feel a need to modify that contract – for instance, to involve themselves in some form of personal growth or encounter, then the contract would need to be renegotiated openly and a consensus achieved before any change was made.

Because the group had many years of social work behind them it was not surprising that while they were eager to learn they were also very conscious of what might be explored in such a group and somewhat defensive of their status as senior professionals. However, the group started well enough on the basis of an exchange of experiences – anecdotal and largely humorous. At this stage they were constantly reminded by the group leader to examine what they saw happening and to modify their total absorption in the content of their interchanges to look at the consequences they were having on them as a group and at the processes that were occurring. Gradually they became more able to see the dynamics of their own behaviour and indeed became absorbed and fascinated by it.

The group comprised four women and three men and for the first weeks the group thawed both to themselves and to the group leader at roughly the same speed, showing much good humour, some anger, some teasing and an ever-growing awareness of the processes they were exploring. About the tenth session, however, there appeared a little tension and some indication that perhaps a change of course was required. In the next session one of the male members opened up the idea that in order for the group to progress further and faster they would have to explore themselves much more than they had done so far. Somewhat surprisingly the rest of the group agreed, with the exception of one of the men. A kind of euphoria about their progress seemed to have overtaken them and their sense of security was founded on this.

The sole dissenter reminded them of their contractual obligation to renegotiate for major change, and stressed the fact that from his observation the group was being swept along by its own success. He warned that several people were not really prepared for such a change and were not really aware of what was involved. At first there was disbelief, and some teasing, but as the rest of the group realised that he was serious the attack started in earnest. What emerged was an enormous degree of hostility. He was accused of never having been serious about the group (he had been one of the more humorous contributors), of sabotaging the group's every effort, of putting people down, of being superior and so on. The victim was quite startled by this attack and made some attempt to pass off the attack and to defend himself. The response was even more overwhelmingly hostile, aggressive and vindictive, bringing not only his behaviour in the group and on the course under fire, but also his personal and professional life.

The leader asked the group to tell him what was happening and was brusquely told that this one man had been ruining the group from the start. As they were now hardly susceptible to a rational approach the leader informed the victim that he thought that he not only had a point to make but an absolute right to make it. At this juncture the leader was undecided as to whether this attack should be stopped, diverted or exposed. In the end he opted for support, reasoning that the basis for the attack was uncertainty about the change that the group had proposed for itself and that this attack was a method of laying those fears off on the resister. Once this process was established the group might be managed out of their hostility and into a lacuna where they would be able to face those fears and bring them out into the open. This would mean that all the hidden agendas around the proposed change could be discussed and a new contract framed.

The basis of this analysis lay on the fact that the scapegoating process was a temporary strategy and, with careful management, would result not only in a negotiated but also in an increased awareness in the group of the pressures, influences and processes which, so far, they had not really looked at.

So the group leader supported the victim, and constantly sought to defuse the group's hostility by pointing out what was happening and by reminding them of their agreement to negotiate change. He also drew on his previous experience of groups to form analogies with the existing situation and was able to use examples from the group's previous sessions.

The first change of direction came when the matter was still not resolved at the end of the session and the leader refused to extend it, a move which was deliberately intended to draw some of the hostility to the leader. This was successful and a heated and brief negotiation was set up which resulted in another session being planned for later the same day. There were now two scapegoats, the leader and the original victim. The leader pointed out that two victims formed a subgroup which was rather more powerful than one isolated group member.

Although the extra session was heated, there were beginning to be signs that other members were having second thoughts about what they were doing and a series of small conflicts began to break out. As the heat diminished by being diffused, the extra group was closed by the leader on the basis that the group was no longer entirely united in blaming the original victim for ruining the group's attempt at progress.

Over the next two sessions a real negotiation was established about the next stage of development and how it should be approached. What emerged quite clearly from this was a remarkable increment in honesty as three members of the group admitted they had felt very threatened by the original proposal to change to personal exposure but had also felt that they could not say so because they would, they felt, have been hindering the group's development, of which they were very proud. So when the original victim had been attacked for doing what they were actually afraid of doing, they joined in with great gusto, relieved that any blame for delaying the group's progress would not be pinned onto them. Of course they felt some guilt about this, and this sharpened and fuelled their attack.

The fortunate result of this was the development of a deeper understanding of the irrational transfer of blame, of the way that transient scapegoating could be managed and how benefit can be derived from the process. One member said: 'I was furious. I thought – all the hard work, all the learning is going to be lost and it's all his fault. What I didn't realise was that I was scared. I felt I had so much I didn't want the others to know about. Now I see that I was more likely to have destroyed the group than "X" that we were all attacking.'

Although this was a very brief episode of scapegoating it was very intense because the fear among the group members of potential loss of self-esteem generated by their professional seniority was very great so it fuelled a very intense and very damaging attack. The supportive, diversionary, delaying and information-giving techniques of the leader maintained the group intact and provided time for the process of rational understanding of what was happening to develop, so that the fears and guilt could be expressed and discharged.

One other situation that would indicate management rather than any attempt to stop the process of scapegoating or to resolve it arises when the element of uniqueness is present. In the experience of Anne (Chapter 6), the purpose of the group in setting her up as a scapegoat depended wholly on the coincidence of the group's failure to organise themselves and Anne being a person who sought confirmation of her own worthless state. Given that the activity in which they were engaged – preparing a dramatic presentation – could be successfully concluded, then the need to blame Anne for everything that went wrong would disappear.

Anne's case displays only partially the kind of pattern where a situation which precipitates a bout of scapegoating is finite, because Anne's particular self-destroying need was very much more a permanent issue and liable to make her a victim in any group which had need to shift blame from themselves to someone else. However, in its pure form a strictly limited situation that is hardly likely to recur is certainly one in which an attempt at management should be made to see the process through to the point where the scapegoating process withers away for lack of any need to continue. This is a somewhat dangerous process in that the assumption of a finite time may be wrong. It is only beneficial if that situation is not only of short duration but also has foci of intervention as, for instance, assessing that the situation can be successfully resolved and providing support to the victim for the period of pressure.

The other danger lies in the fact that if the group continues in existence after a successful completion of the situation that was fuelling the scapegoating, there is always the possibility that another crisis may precipitate victimisation of the same member on the basis of past memory, whether the precipitating situation is similar to the first one or not. In short, the original victim may have tacitly acquired in the collective memory the role of useful scapegoat.

As in all management of the process, when the crisis is past it is almost always advisable to review what happened, why and the aftermath. The chance to expose the mechanics of the process should never be missed because once they become part of the awareness of the group an element of choice is introduced which did not previously exist. It may not be possible to create alternative methods of coping with group tension and frustration, but at least a situation can be created in which warning signals can be noted and a common language of explanation provided for future occasions if necessary.

Management is to be seen not as condoning scapegoating but as a strategy which, given the intensity and sudden development of the process, seeks to limit the damage that can occur and to ensure a relatively profitable outcome. Now we must turn our attention to the process of not controlling alone but of resolving so that a new process of dealing with threat, fear, guilt, obstruction and frustration can be designed and made operational. Thus, from management, which is in essence a tiding-over process, we must now turn our attention to those indicators of the need for, and the possibility of, a process of resolution, of turning the process of scapegoating into different channels and of creating an understanding of the process and hence of developing a choice of how to proceed.

Chapter 10

The resolution of scapegoating

Scapegoating, for example, has been posited on the one hand to be a resultant of group efforts to foster or maintain group integration, and on the other to be primarily a consequence of the specific provocations, deviant behaviors or ineptness of scapegoated individuals.

(Feldman 1969: 30–1)

Throughout this book I have maintained a distinction between the purposes of scapegoating, as manifested by the scapegoater's needs and actions, and the attributes and needs of the victims, the scapegoats. It is possible to show that the two main thrusts of attempts to deal with the problems caused by scapegoating maintain this distinction. Indeed, Feldman, in the article quoted above, also wrote:

Accordingly group workers should be able to intervene in such processes at either the individual or group level insofar as discrete, accessible, and potent focuses for intervention come to be delineated.

where the individual referred to is the scapegoat victim and the group is the scapegoating agency.

The processes to which Feldman refers in this quotation are of course those of scapegoating. He is suggesting that it is possible to intervene in that process both at the group level and at an individual level which, by implication, means tackling both scapegoaters and their victims. But before we pursue this idea and others from different sources concerning the resolution of scapegoating we must start by discussing what differences need to exist which essentially influence the choice of resolution rather than management.

The major selection factors for management were the sudden onset of the process; a perception of the dangers inherent in trying to stop or change what was happening; the essentially transient nature of the process; and the possibility of an excess of benefit both for group and individual over damage – in sum, that the exercise of control and damage limitation was not only essential but the methodology of choice.

I have already indicated that scapegoating seldom if ever occurs in the early stages of a group. The sole important exception to this in my own experience has been the formation of a new group which contained members of a previous group that had recently ceased to exist. The group members had a considerable degree of unfinished business with one another, which included a large amount of blame for the collapse of the previous group.

As this was a rather unusual situation I shall continue to assert that it is the norm for scapegoating to take place only when a group has been in existence for some time – indeed long enough for difficulties to emerge for which no obvious causes are discoverable and for those characteristics of certain members to emerge which will serve to focus the scapegoating process when it occurs. Because of the time scapegoating takes to develop, any attempt to resolve it already has evidence of that development and of the potential of some members to be victims as an indication of the form resolution should take.

The first hurdle must, as always, be that of recognition. It is essential that group leaders should be reasonably clear in their own minds that the process which the group is operating is one of blame transfer and that the basic ingredient of a lack of 'real' justification is obviously present. Some writers argue that it is seldom possible to know the real causes of scapegoating because of the irrational nature of the process and because of the unknown and unknowable emotional and thought processes of those involved. But such authors also state that to know what causes a process is not a necessary condition of being able to do something about it, as the behavioural consequences are plain for all to see. I would not dispute this assertion about the difficulty of knowing causes, and I am well aware that causes are often attributed on the basis of theoretical belief rather than on any provable factual evidence of existence. Nevertheless, the point remains that similar patterns of behaviour that are clearly visible may stem from extremely different causes, and at least it would be politic and intelligent to make some attempt to discover the cause of overt and critical blame-laying behaviour irrespective of whether or not what is being observed stems from rational suspicion that the subject is either materially or collaterally responsible for the group's predicament.

Most writers agree that in cases of true scapegoating – that is, when the individual who is blamed for some event is not actually responsible for its occurrence – the actual process is preceded by an increasing bewilderment, frustration and anger on the part of group members. They are aware that something is wrong; indeed they most frequently state this as a categorical fact and often enough they discuss what is wrong. But in many such instances they tend to locate the problem in areas of group life or in outside factors which essentially have little to do with the actual problem. Diagnostically this sequence is important. It starts with vague assertions of dissatisfaction with the group's progress, proceeds to specific complaints, which are then followed by the application of a remedy. Usually, however, this 'remedy' does not even supply a temporary relief, except that which comes along with the very transient feeling of success stemming from an awareness of having made an attempt.

Feldman and Wodarski (1975: 89) are among those writers who suggest that, as it may be impossible or even useless to elicit the causes of scapegoating behaviour, treatment should focus on the current conditions which sustain it at both individual and group levels. In the process of assessing whether a scapegoating situation exists, it is suggested that the following information should be sought:

- Which of the victim's behaviours or aspects of personality constitutes the provocation for scapegoating or sustains the behaviour when established, and in what way does the victim react to the scapegoating process? [The authors suggest that the victim's reactions to being scapegoated are very important because they frequently serve to reinforce the scapegoating behaviour.]
- How do the scapegoat and his or her peers regard the problems?
- What information about the scapegoat's background, family, school, job, etc., is available and relevant?

- What similar information about the other members of the group is also available and relevant?
- What information is available about the scapegoat as a member of the present group and about the other members, particularly in relation to roles and the structure of power, status and communication within the group?

Based upon this information, or upon as much of it as can be collected, the authors indicate that the 'dynamic nature of those social forces involved in the scapegoating behaviour will be apparent'. Normally I would regard this as a very sanguine statement, but all the evidence of my own experience and of many other groupworkers would seem to indicate that without even so much historical evidence as Feldman and Wodarski would have us collect, the process of scapegoating seems to be remarkably obvious when it occurs. It may be the pattern of one opposed and attacked by the many; it may be that the process of off-loading badness is common to our experience; but whatever it is, recognition, at least in a small group, is seldom difficult to achieve.

The next part of the scapegoating process is that someone within the group's ambit – not necessarily a member of the group but almost certainly connected with it in some way – becomes the focus of blame and attack. Members of management, particularly those responsible for the oversight of several small, relatively autonomous professional groups, are frequently selected as scapegoats in large organisations. In these cases the essential factor of recognition between the 'real' cause and an 'irrational' cause is frequently very difficult to determine as management certainly does create situations which, far from freeing others to operate within clearly defined bounds, succeed in hampering and confining their best efforts. Equally, professional units with a greatly overestimated value placed upon their independence within the organisation of which they are part, not infrequently invoke exactly the management response of which they complain.

Studies of teams have often revealed that the true causes of frustration and complaint which are laid at the door of inefficient management can be located in team members' inability to assess for themselves the degree of independent responsibility they have been accorded by the system, and an equal inability to programme their activities to meet new demands. The latter, strangely enough, is often based upon an expectation that a large organisation will actually generate the procedures within which such units can work.

Irrespective of the actual reason, context or choice of victim, if the process of scapegoating gets underway in a gradual fashion then the basic element for determining the choice of resolution is in place.

The characteristics of potential scapegoats, the group's developmental stage and any overt provocation, should have been registered by the group leader. Essentially, scapegoating is a harmful ploy and unless a group is cynically or desperately prepared to exploit and punish some of its own members in order to secure the temporary survival of the rest, then it is a tactic which needs to be exposed for what it is and, at best, the causes of the need to blame must be discovered and dealt with. At second best a less damaging form of coping should be devised and implemented as an alternative.

I propose to look at some widely accepted and used formulations for dealing with the process of scapegoating and to suggest that the obvious similarities indicate the possible presence of common guidelines.

Northen (1969) suggested the following ideas:

- Attempt to prepare the ground for the clarification and analytical processes by encouraging members to participate more fully under supportive guidance.
- Clarify the conditions which led to scapegoating.
- Analyse the stresses within a group that result in the projection of hostility onto a victim.
- Analyse the provocative characteristics of the chosen scapegoat.
- Confront members with their inclination to stereotype others as occurs in scapegoating.

These are broad techniques which are applied, as Feldman suggested, to both the group members as scapegoaters and to the individual victim, though the main weight is given to the former. The problem with this kind of approach is that there is a bland assumption that the processes of clarification and analysis are easy to apply and that the basic stresses will reveal themselves without a great deal of effort. If this were the case then there is a distinct possibility that scapegoating would never take place, for any group would soon have discovered for themselves what were the roots of their problems and promptly devised some way to cope, even if it was to ask for help. But they would have known!

Consider the complexity of these processes of locating and reducing stress; of discovering the predisposing causes of scapegoating as revealed in the following example offered by Ken Heap (1977: 155–63) in *Group Theory for Social Workers*.

Heap uses the cases of Elisabeth (whom we have met before), Michael and Anne and presents the techniques that were used in each instance.

In all three cases intervention was clearly directed to giving support to the whole group, which involved the groupworker in *active support* and *unequivocal acceptance* of the group members' impulses and the feelings which aroused guilt. The result of such intervention was to markedly decrease the level of anxiety in the group and to refocus the liberated energy away from the scapegoat and onto the process of considering how they might deal directly with their feelings rather than through the process of projecting them onto a selected victim.

The victims in these cases were relieved of the pressure of being under humiliating attack, and thus also freed from their role entrapment and able to seek for other and more mature relationships with their colleagues.

Heap comments that the role of the worker is crucial in this developmental sequence in promoting (a) the prototype of an understanding rather than a condemning adult figure, (b) a role model of an approach to dealing with problems from a base of reality rather than from one of anxiety and fantasy, and (c) a basis of understanding through better information of the formation and power of feelings and impulses.

All three of Heap's examples were of groups of young people in which the general problems of adolescence, common in 1977, motivated the scapegoating procedure. In Elisabeth's case the situation may well have been helped by a three-months absence during which time her group, with help, were able to assess its methods of coping with its problems. Heap ends his discussion of these three problems with a concern about the situation when the scapegoat has a 'pathological' need to be a victim, which, in his estimation, requires outside help. Thus treatment is seen as a contribution ' . . . aimed not at protection, not at mediation, not at judgment of the scapegoat, but at relief of the feelings of guilt, deviance, inadequacy, fear of isolation or whatever qualities arouse the need for projection and expiation'.

An analysis of the treatment programmes offered to these three groups reveals the following:

1. *Recognition*: It is axiomatic that no attempt to cope with scapegoating which is producing difficulties within a group can be put in place until there is a clear recognition not just that scapegoating is happening but also of the situation from which it derives its energy.

2. *Removal of the victim*: In Elisabeth's case this was not set in motion by the groupworker but by the arrival of a family crisis. However, it illustrates the point that the absence of the victim on a temporary basis gives an opportunity for the group to explore what it was actually doing and why. Thus temporary removal of the victim may be considered as a technique that can be deliberately employed, given that the removed victim can be given adequate attention during the period of absence. Total removal without being able to concentrate on the problem within the group stands to create a reassertion of the scapegoating behaviour with a newly selected victim, because the underlying motivation to blame, to project, to sacrifice and to ease unacknowledged discomfort still remains active.

3. *The role of the groupworker*: The most effective techniques were:
   (a) providing a role model of an understanding, non-condemnatory adult;
   (b) being a source of accurate information about revealed problems and of methods of coping with them;
   (c) exposing what was happening in the group and pointing up consequences and choices without bias or coercive pressure, for example,
      (i) accepting 'badness' and thus bringing it out into the open and making it discussable;
      (ii) highlighting provocation and the response patterns it produced, revealing that the relationship between stimulus and response was not irrevocably fixed;
      (iii) highlighting the needs of the scapegoats, especially their apparent need for confirmation of themselves as bad or worthless.

The whole process, based upon the initial recognition, has been to insert some rational consideration between stimulus and response, an act made possible only by some clearly visible change in circumstances like Elisabeth's absence or by the deliberate intervention to introduce the possibility of new insights.

4. *The analysis of the victim's needs*: It has always been an accepted truism that removal of maladaptive modes of need satisfaction must be accompanied or followed by the implanting and use of new and more adaptive modes. The greater the need for confirmation of badness, for instance, the more urgent it becomes to cope with that need in a more acceptable way or to reduce its force when one source of supplying it has been removed. There are some similiarities in this process with forms of psychological addiction.

It is interesting in this context that MacLennan and Felsenfeld, whose notes on the scapegoating process in groups of adolescents we looked at earlier, put such great emphasis on selecting out possible scapegoats when the group is being formed. This is a suggestion which implies that the characteristics of potential victims are not only well known but also easily recognised.

Of course, given the fact that obvious difference is one of the prime requirements of a victim, the process of selecting may not be as difficult as it would appear. But there is clearly the great probability of being wrong for the simple reason that different aspects of difference are potential foci for different kinds of group problem.

In groupwork literature the classic analysis of scapegoating and of the methods of resolving the process are to be found in a paper by Garland and Kolodny (1966). After discussing the basic theoretical concepts relating to the process, and suggesting that resolution is usually to be made along the lines of pursuing changes in group structure, attempts to change the scapegoaters, tension-reduction techniques, diversionary tactics, cut-offs and bypassing, they offer the following compendium of techniques of coping for group leaders:

- The procedure is squashed by the group leader.
- The composition of the group is changed.
- Information about the situation is fed into the group.
- The scapegoat is protected by the leader.
- A diversion is created.
- An attempt is made to reduce interaction.

- The group is supported and given the opportunity to discharge its hostility.
- An attempt is made to clarify the motivations behind the scapegoating.
- Some attempt is made to focus on the constructive value that the scapegoat has for the group.
- The group can be encouraged to control the scapegoat by containing his or her provocative behaviour without actually scapegoating.
- By the use of role play, other members can learn what is involved.
- The scapegoat can be removed from the group.

We have already encountered several of these techniques both in discussion and in some of the examples. They tend to suffer from the same factors as the Northen list, e.g. by being too broad and in seeming to believe that by saying that something is a good procedure that this is the same as indicating how it shall be performed. Also the collection is an indiscriminate list of approaches which do not have much direct connection with the many different kinds of group situations in which scapegoating tends to occur. The Heap example, on the other hand, offers precise targeting of techniques with probably one of the most difficult methods to use successfully, that of the removal of the scapegoat from the group. The problem with this technique is that it looks like a surprisingly simple and obvious solution and clearly based upon concern for the victim, but it rarely results in a long-term solution for two good and obvious reasons.

First, removing the scapegoat does nothing to deal with the reasons why a victim was considered to be necessary. It merely exacerbates the situation by removing the possibility of a temporary release from tension. Second, and following on from the first reason, because the problem still remains it is almost inevitable that, unless guided to another kind of solution, the group will seek a replacement scapegoat from either the remaining members or some close affiliate of the group. What appears easy and logical on the surface is seldom lastingly effective. This is not to say that there are no actual situations where, for the safety of the scapegoat, it is essential that he or she should be removed from the group, but usually only after the probability of control and management discussed in the last chapter have been considered and rejected as inappropriate.

At this point it is perhaps necessary to try to introduce further clarity into the probable approaches to the resolution of scapegoating.

Having dealt with the problem of recognition, about which incidentally scant reference will be found in the literature on scapegoating – probably on the somewhat mistaken assumption that the difference between scapegoating and accusation is obvious – there are only three areas of approach, i.e. to the cause or problem, to the process and to the victim. We shall now consider what is available in each of these three areas.

CAUSE OR PROBLEM

With the solitary exception which occurs, as in public scapegoating, when the process of the deflection of blame is a conscious and deliberate strategy of evasion, the major problem of deciding cause is that it is almost always hidden, or at least unsuspected. It cannot be stressed too often that this basic ingredient of obscurity is the main factor in precipitating the scapegoating process. It tends to be observed as bewilderment and frustration. There is some understanding that things have gone wrong – a feeling that is powerful and creates tension, but has no immediately obvious focus. Human beings seem to be more or less incapable of accepting the inexplicable, and if no realistic proof – i.e. having some logical explanation for events that are emotional, behavioural or situational – is forthcoming, then explanations are concocted in order to relieve the cognitive dissonance of there being an event with no logical explanation. Thus scapegoating takes place. It is a form of explanation.

There are two basic approaches to the problem of cause, both based upon the fact or belief that when the true causes of tension are revealed and when the real causes, as opposed to the concocted ones, are available for inspection, then there is a possibility that they can be dealt with. The first of the two approaches, which are not mutually exclusive, uses the theoretical guidelines and attempts to match the observed facts to the concepts – in other words, to use generalised but structured ideas to illuminate a particular incident. The second approach regards the individual event of scapegoating as being relatively unique and explores it in an effort to describe it.

There are several comments to make about these approaches. In the first instance they are both exploratory and such a process needs at least the presence of two major factors to have any chance of being even remotely successful. These are (1) time and (2) at least a basic willingness on the part of the group members to become involved. Where neither of these is available in adequate degree, the preferred option for intervention is one of management (see Chapter 9) rather than resolution. It must also be stressed that any investigation of causes is usually more effective in its execution rather than any ultimate decision that may be reached; that is, the process tends to be rather more rewarding than any outcome.

In Chapter 7 a discussion of the various theoretical approaches was presented so that it should serve now just to recall them briefly if only to discover not only the obscurity they describe but also their probable complexity.

- Frustration, aggression and displacement
- Projection and psychic discomfort
- General hostility
- The personal characteristics of scapegoaters – the authoritarian personality
- Conscious avoidance and victim choice
- Deflection – a rational defensive measure
- Protection of self-esteem
- Attribution theory
- The dislike hypothesis
- Propinquity, availability and restricted choice
- Situational factors.

As I have stressed before, this is a mixed bag of concepts, some of which are as relevant to the choice of victim as they are to the energising of the process. However, they can operate as guidelines. The important factor, of course, is the actual observational acuity of the person who uses them as a method of seeking to bring out into the open the power springs behind the group's actions. There is evidence that the theoretical ideas which eventually appear to fit the individual case are of less importance to group members than the fact that they have been given a language (of a sort), which offers the opportunity to search out and describe what was previously obscure and without means of being expressed. When it becomes possible to talk about something in words that are commonly understood among those directly involved, then this is almost always accompanied by some sense that an element of control has been created that did not previously exist.

Given that this element of control can be achieved, then one major step towards reducing the blind assault on a relatively innocent victim can take place. But it is clear that however convinced a group leader may be of the efficacy in explanation of any particular approach, it must remain essentially true that, at best, such explanations are just that, a language or a set of symbols which allow for a degree of logical control of the basic patterns of behaviour which the group is producing. Thus, for example, if rational strategy is apparent in the process, what need is there to seek for other factors, at least in the initial stages?

The second approach in this area of seeking for causes is based upon either the absence of clues that would indicate the use of one or more of the theoretical guidelines, or an assumption that there is no good purpose in attempting to discover causes but to deal with what is much more obvious and readily at hand, namely the consequences. Thus disclosure in this case centres around discussion of a description of what is happening and a conscious search for why it is occurring. If this only reveals a large degree of frustration and puzzlement, then much has been gained for at least it stands revealed that the scapegoating has no clear or even logical basis.

Another point about the search for causes is that it can be self-defeating in several ways. For instance, it can become the sole preoccupation of the group members to the neglect of their original purposes and it can also contribute to the avoidance of actually doing something about any causes that are discovered. When discussion of causes takes place on the basis of a discrete event in a particular group, then although the causes may never be clearly elucidated, the group's tramlined processes of thinking are often abandoned in favour of new approaches – and new thinking, or perhaps even just thinking, is introduced into the situation.

One cause that can be exposed quite readily if evidence is available concerns the personalities of the scapegoaters. Though such exposure is a relatively easy thing to achieve, it must be remembered that personal characteristics in, say, the form of an authoritarian personality are not primary causes. They are the factors which shape the response of an individual to the experience of frustration, bewilderment and guilt. This is also true of the factors of face-saving and of intense personal dislike. Thus, in one sense we should consider them as part of the scapegoating process, but because they are not essential parts of the actual act but constitute what can be called 'predisposing factors', I consider that they are better placed under the rubric of cause.

The process of exposure is perhaps best attempted by example, if possible, from previous occurrences which demonstrate the effect of the personality factors involved. As usual, in dealing with predisposing factors, their exposure and acceptance may well cause the process of scapegoating in the particular situation under review to cease. But although it may also make group members more aware of their predisposition to blame others, it does little or nothing to expose and deal with the actual cause. The main function of this form of exposure must lie in promoting the idea that it will be necessary to design different ways of coping with tension, stress, guilt, etc., and to prepare warning signals for the emergence of the predisposing behaviour. It is similar to being prepared to minimise storm damage and to have the equipment and help to deal with it when it arrives, there being no way to deal with the actual causes.

PROCESS

In discussing the process of creating a scapegoat, Garvin (1981:99) says 'the worker should try to prevent some members from becoming locked into such roles in early meetings as it is difficult to remove a deviant label once it has been affixed'.

So, on the assumption frequently expressed by writers of the universality of the scapegoating process, Garvin's suggestion makes sense. In action it would involve, first, giving information to the group about the high degree of probability of the occurrence of scapegoating; and, second, when there are signs that individuals in the group are apparently setting up such a procedure, to point to what is happening before group members become 'locked into' their appropriate scapegoating roles.

The main approach to the resolution of scapegoating which is directed at the process itself is once more that of making commonly visible what is happening, and, when some consensus about the situation is available, attempting to describe what the probable consequences will be. This must be done as impartially and as objectively as possible so that the next stage – which is to ask the question about those probable consequences, i.e. 'Is this what you want to happen?' – is not seen as a threat but as a genuine enquiry about intent.

'Why are you doing this to X?' often elicits answers that are demonstrably non-relevant. Thus, when asked how the group intended to achieve an outcome by the attack on X, the process of providing even a rationalisation tends to reveal a glaring discrepancy between feelings and action – between the tension and the lack of clear knowledge of cause and the actions taken to diminish the dissonance.

Cowger (1979) listed five basic principles for dealing with conflict in a group which, with some slight modification, can form a sound basis for dealing with the actual process of scapegoating. After all, in a very true sense scapegoating is a form of conflict between the scapegoaters and their victim.

The first principle states the absolute necessity of confronting the scapegoaters and the scapegoat with their behaviour. It has already been suggested that this is of the utmost importance and is essentially the first thing that should be done for several reasons.

It is most revealing in group situations to discover how unaware group members are of the actions they are taking. Essentially they know something is happening; they may even actively participate in those happenings; but there is almost always some considerable discrepancy of the understanding of what is happening from individual to individual. Confrontation forces everyone to face those discrepancies and discover if there is any common ground.

Then, again, confrontation actually brings the process itself to a halt while talking about it takes place. Scapegoating is such a universal phenomenon that few group members actually question it or its validity as a group event. Confrontation disrupts this view of the process as one that is 'natural' and therefore acceptable. It tends to reveal the fact that few people in a group have any clear idea why they are attacking one of their peers until they are actually faced with an actual occurrence. Conversely, allowing scapegoating to proceed in the hope that it will go away with no attempt at management or resolution will merely serve to reinforce the belief that it is a 'natural' process and can be operated as and when necessary. This is especially true if the process is actually successful, or even if it only temporarily removes stress and frustration from the group.

Cowger's second principle involved the avoidance of intervening in such a way that a win/lose situation was created. In the context of scapegoating this can be seen as saving either the scapegoat at the expense of the rest of the group, or the group at the cost of sacrificing the scapegoat. The balance of intervention has therefore to be continually adjusted as the situation changes, which is why the simple idea of protecting the scapegoat, however necessary, is seldom wholly satisfactory unless it is accompanied by other strategies which are less biased in favour of one side of the issue.

Certainly a heavy-handed put-down of either side will result in a drastic loss of motivation and commitment to the group and will often create an image of power being applied in a biased way. In general, the overall effect will be to make the group's existence much more fragile.

The themes of bias, legitimacy and fairness in the exercise of power are continued into another of Cowger's principles, which is concerned with what might be called even-handedness. Cowger describes this as the worker maintaining relationships with the *whole* group. Of course there is always a tendency when such situations as scapegoating arise to concentrate attention on the main protagonists. But scapegoating is a whole-group phenomenon in its effects, if not in its initiation and projection. While the main activists no doubt require considerable attention, the processes of adjustment, confrontation, explanation and discussion are essentially whole-group activities. It is the problem of the whole group and the resolution is likewise the concern of all members.

Inevitably another of Cowger's principles states that the process should be clarified and integrated. This can probably be accepted as important without further comment. The author then makes his final statement, which is that standards and ground rules should be set and norms developed.

This is indeed a very crucial process. If we are to assume that the initial causes of the need to lay blame, frustration, etc., onto a victim are not accessible – or even if they are, that there is not much chance that they can be eliminated and therefore the need to discharge tension will arise again – then to devise rules of engagement is probably the best strategy of intervention that can be formulated.

It is axiomatic that one of the basic drives behind scapegoating lies as much in a secondary frustration as in the primary one. In most cases the secondary annoyance comes into force when individuals and groups are aware of their anger and bad feeling, but have not the slightest idea what to do about them. Usually previous experience has laid in a programme for dealing with matters of this nature which, while it may have been only marginally successful on previous applications, is all that individuals have. Given the human tendency explored here to blame someone, anyone, in order to evade responsibility, punishment or other consequence, it is not surprising that this tendency forms the basis for most responses to frustration.

What is being proposed here is that the tendency to blame is accepted as normal, or at least ubiquitous, and thus there is a need to explore ways in which it can be expressed which do not necessarily involve a probably innocent victim, chosen on the basis of differences that have little or no reference to the actual problem. This involves the proposal, discussion and acceptance by the group of a set of procedural rules which provide a rational alternative to victimisation. Basically such rules should give a clear indication that when levels of frustration and difficulty arise within the group, every member has an absolute right, if not a duty, to signal that he or she is distressed and to make available to everyone else the nature of that distress whatever its vagueness, uncertainty or lack of focus of origin. Concomitantly the group will also have a rule which states that the members have a responsibility to pay attention to this kind of statement however peculiar it may seem, and acord it adequate consideration.

This is not easy to do, and cannot be done at all if the trust levels within the group are low. Group leaders must therefore use their discretion about the degree of intensity with which such rules are proposed, discussed and accepted. Rules have no validity whatsoever if they define a behavioural standard well beyond the capacity of group members to achieve. If the rules are successfully activated and prevent scapegoating taking place, then they will tend to become numbered among the norms of the group. The problems which actually activated the scapegoating process originally will still exist, but at least a functional method of discharge will be in place which should help the group to concentrate its energies on the main tasks for which it was created.

This approach ignores causes but can also be combined with such an approach if the appropriate clues are available. However, it stands as an effective method in its own right centred on the 'here and now' of the group and serves to initiate discussion of what the group is actually seeking to achieve by setting in motion the process of scapegoating and may also bring into the arena of discussion some consideration of why.

VICTIM

In Chapter 8 some of the theoretical concepts about the scapegoats, the victims, were listed. In brief it contained the following:

- Social powerlessness
- Dislike
- Personal characteristics: behaviour patterns, provocative behaviour, attention seeking, deviance
- Difference.

The strategies of resolution in the area of the victim are once again concerned with exposure – that is, in showing that a victim has been chosen not because of any real responsibility for what ails the group but because of some of the factors listed above. This is to employ a change of perception gambit which goes from irrational belief in a member's responsibility to an understanding of the true nature of the basis of selection.

Another change of perception gambit is concerned with value. It is axiomatic that scapegoats are often members of peripheral value to the group. If that low value rating can be increased, then the probability of that individual being chosen as scapegoat is somewhat reduced.

A situational change can be brought about if the scapegoat can be encouraged to change some aspects of his or her behaviour. However, if that behaviour is essential to the individual's basic needs, then this is much less of a realistic option unless different and less sacrificial ways of satisfaction can be substituted.

It was stated in Chapter 7 that one of the main factors of selection of a scapegoat was the perception by the scapegoaters that their intended victim was most unlikely to be able to present an effective defence or to retaliate. Thus one of the prime ploys in this area of resolution is concerned with the powerlessness of the victim. Assuming that all strategies that do not have as their basic intent the exposure of the actual causes of the scapegoating process but are remedies applied to symptoms, then a strategy which deals with powerlessness has the merit of limiting possible hurt to the victim and possibly of ensuring that he or she no longer becomes a victim in the future. It also gives the group pause for thought about the ethics of attacking its weaker members.

All strategies which aim to expose the group members to information about the victim and their treatment of that selected individual follow somewhat similar paths, and the principles set out by Cowger, discussed earlier, are equally applicable here.

One particular problem that arises in this area of focus has been defined as the victim. This problem lies in the possibility of there being some element of voluntary sacrifice.

I have discussed elsewhere the ubiquitous description of scapegoats as innocent victims and have shown that, while some are not innocent, their complicity in the situation that has generated accusation and opprobrium is usually less than that of the person who deflects the attacks onto them. But the literature on modern scapegoating is essentially clear: there are individuals who deliberately display some or all of those characteristics that are most likely to attract a hostile response when the group is meeting a period of frustration and/or difficulty or a fragile adaptation to changed circumstances.

Garvin (1981:99) suggests that leaders should try to prevent members becoming 'locked into' scapegoat roles; he also suggests that workers can 'promote a group norm that members should take responsibility for their actions towards each other'. Others suggest that individuals with provocative behaviour patterns, attention-seeking needs and other sacrificial tendencies should be selected out of groups.

That such a process has to be based upon some considerable prior knowledge of potential group members seems to eliminate it as a method of dealing with the particular aspect of being a scapegoat. Once more the essential process of exposing what is happening is obviously necessary, and is the beginning of a process in which the attention needs of such individuals can probably be supplied without recourse to martyrdom. If this latter kind of need has become a pathological one, then unless the group is especially attuned to dealing with personality disorders of this magnitude it would be essential that option number 12, in Garland and Kolodny's list, should be operated and the individual removed from the group.

A particularly useful paper on dealing with the problem of personal dislike as a focal attractor of scapegoating activities was presented by Feldman in 1969. He believed that those who were intensely disliked group members 'tend to be characterised by a pattern of social attributes that contribute to the development and/or maintenance of their unique social position' (p. 37). In other words, their behaviour in groups reinforced and maintained the dislike already felt for them by their peers and heightened the possibility that in any time of group stress they would be selected as targets for scapegoating.

As Feldman saw, the main components of this reinforcing behaviour lay in the individual's presentation to the group of a 'low commitment to group norms, inadequate performance of important group functions, low liking for peers and low social power'. Feldman's suggested approach was not so much to make these properties visible but to work directly with the individual and the group to change both the individual's presentation and the group's perception of it. For instance, he commented that a low commitment to group norms could possibly be changed by making clearer what was involved, reinforcing or rewarding the conformity of the disliked member to those norms and in reducing the power of the group's sanctions for non-conformity.

The performance of important group functions can be enhanced by direct instruction for the disliked member in the methods of achieving success; and activities within the group can be programmed to demonstrate such skills and abilities that the disliked member possesses. With regard to a low level of popularity, Feldman suggest that as this is often based on a lack of adequate knowledge about an individual the group should be encouraged to greater social interaction and communication with each other; goals should be set for the group which can actually be achieved by cooperative effort and procedures should be instituted which 'assure recognition and acceptance of the legitimate rights and powers of all members'.

As with all interventions directed at the scapegoat victims, Feldman's indirect approach, away from the process of scapegoating but towards redefining the potential victims, is a deliberate choice and ignores the probable deep-seated causes. Indeed, Feldman writes that his available data 'will not permit empirical examination of causal relationships'. It is my opinion also that the main value of attempting to use theoretical concepts to allocate causes to the intial impetus towards scapegoating is that it provides a language and a set of concepts to discuss what might be happening rather than a description of actual events, psychic or physical. Dealing with the process as it occurs in the context of a particular group and/or with the victims of the process is largely pragmatic in nature, and although it may be a symptomatic approach it can form the basis of a damage limitation exercise and does procure the time that will allow for the development of procedures necessary to promote alternative and less potentially damaging forms of discharging tension.

Chapter 11

Rite, ritual or survival strategy?
Final considerations

Garland and Kolodny (1966), after their researches into the process of scapegoating, decided that the process violated every ethical tenet to which most modern societies subscribed. They pointed out that it was one of the most universally found forms of group event and, because of this, tends to be accepted as inevitable, including whatever the consequences of the process may be. Indeed, most of us accept it as part of everyday experience.

Such is the ubiquitous nature of the scapegoating process.

The current rational approach to social problems, while proving very effective in some areas, has been woefully inadequate in others. In essence, it has been least successful in those areas of human existence which are inhabited by fear. Although people will offer reasonable explanations for certain kinds of behaviour, the explanations that are offered in many cases are of the nature of good or bad fortune, or of a belief in the ability of remote astral bodies to influence human behaviour, or of the need to hedge one's bets with lucky charms, talismanic objects, etc., all of which would seem to demonstrate that, reasonable or not, the modern man is still a creature who implicitly believes in mystical forces of some kind, but who may find it very difficult to admit to these beliefs in the face of the very strong current trends of rational explanation.

Joseph Campbell (1973) believed that myths were an essential part of humanity's equipment, indeed he called one of his books *Myths to Live By*. Of course he knew that myths have no objective reality; that as explanations of physical history they were false. But he also believed that the mythic imagination was a fact of the human mind.

There is not much to dispute in this belief, but the method by which myths are expressed must be characteristic of the period in which they are used. In the twentieth century, evil is no longer regarded as some potent force existing in its own right and is only commonly spoken about as a form of emphasis, as when President Reagan referred to the Soviet Union as the 'Evil Empire'. The methods of coping with it have also changed from ritual to attempts to change individual patterns of behaviour, and from magic and ritual, designed to pass the tangible evil onto others, to the carefully calculated process in public scapegoating of setting up others to take the blame – in essence, trying to evade responsibility.

Nevertheless, this in no way says that the basic sensation of fear is any less potent now than it was thousands of years ago. The difference lies not in the basic motivations to action but in the processes which are considered adequate to deal with them.

The main differences between ancient and modern versions of the scapegoating process lie in the comparative complexity of the societies in which the process occurs. Thus, complexity arises in modern societies by the enormously increased numbers and diversities of people involved, with no simple overriding code of conduct or belief, no plain and obvious behaviour that is endorsed by all. Indeed, so complex is modern society and so internally fragmented with so many interests often at odds with one another within its boundaries, that the fact that some behaviour patterns, such as scapegoating, have not only survived but apparently flourished, would seem to indicate that scapegoating serves a very basic human need.

However, when the process is not one in which clear and deliberate intent to deflect censure and punishment is employed, then its roots must lie in some confusion and in some ignorance of the actual causes of frustration and difficulty.

CAUSES

When attempting to discover the causes of social events there is the great problem of the indistinct relationship between cause and effect which occurs so often. The problem is increased by such situations as the distance between two events or the multiplicity of factors involved. In cases at law the attempt to ascertain what actually happened in, say, a criminal event is beset with enormous problems, not the least of which is the subjective nature of evidence, so that although it is always stated that what is being sought is factual truth, what is always established is a level of probability of an occurrence which is directly related to the quality and availability of the evidence.

For instance, if a man walking along a street comes to a corner and in turning around it he bumps into another person coming in the opposite direction, who is to blame? Who was not taking sufficient care; who was preoccupied, in a hurry, not able to see clearly, feeling ill and so on? Given time and an expert eliciting of the evidence in such a simple and direct sequence, the extenuating circumstances could perhaps be laid bare. But time is not available in many circumstances and the blame for such an incident may not be based upon any reasoned assessment of what was involved.

When someone is held responsible for the collapse of a business there is a maze of indistinct and complex relationships between that individual's behaviour and the consequent collapse. Indeed, the necessity to blame something or someone in an organisation where the paths of responsibility are shared, cross, recross, are delegated and accepted in a multitude of ways, makes it almost impossible to establish irrefutable links between a given person and the eventual collapse. It is also relatively much easier to involve others and to spread the confusion with reference to other circumstances and thus to introduce doubt. With care this activity can be taken to the point of absolving the original (and probably the actual) culprit and to the setting up of others – a process that is not as easy in smaller face-to-face groups.

To some extent there is always some obscurity about the causes of events, or at least there is a high degree of ambiguity. People often know that something is wrong or is going astray, but they do not have any clear idea of what or why. Someone or something must be causing the problems, but as they may be involved in the situation themselves, most immediate observers have a reduced probability of being clear about causes. It is no accident that knowledgeable outsiders have a clearer vision of the problems of an organisation than do any of its members.

There is, apparently, a very strong urge for members of an organisation to give a name to what they think is happening. By so doing they create a strong feeling that, to a certain extent, they understand the problem. Thus to blame someone or something for what is happening equally tends to produce a sense of having solved the problem of cause. In the relief which follows, those involved can convince themselves that they can now forget the problem and get on with what they should be doing. However, in many cases the real cause of the problem has not been isolated.

Despite this, the sense of satisfaction may continue because one of the two major methods of dealing with such problems has been operated, i.e. perception of the nature of the problem has been changed, but the other, changing the actual circumstances causing the problem, is still unused.

It is through this process that many people in organisations are sacrificed on the belief that they are causing problems, when indeed the problems are elsewhere and often reappear after the sacrifice has been made. Sometimes this is a quite deliberate process because the real problems cannot be discovered or because they may be known but are commonly accepted as insoluble. Then a process is created of scapegoating someone just to produce a semblance of coping with the problems, and this frequently secures a transient reprieve because others believe that the problems have been dealt with.

LINGERING SUPERSTITION

When lightning struck York minster causing a fire which destroyed a large part of that ancient church many people were unable to accept that this was a wholly natural occurrence. In the daily papers of the time the utterances of the newly created Bishop of Durham, which were considerably at variance with what many church people would have expected from a bishop, were actually advanced as the reason for the partial destruction of York minster. It was suggested that the bishop's pronouncements on some central issues of Christian belief were of such a scandalous and shocking nature that God had demonstrated his displeasure by causing the lightning to strike and burn part of the roof of the minster.

The distinction between a cause and its subsequent effect – which are directly related though sometimes complex – and events which are in no real sense related, is frequently very confusing and presupposes a whole series of connections between apparently unrelated events which have a different order of existence or belief to that which one would consider 'normal'. One of the most important of these 'different' factors is time, which also inhabits the normal world, and this adds to the confusion. For instance, an event which precipitates another obviously precedes it in time, often very closely. It is therefore very easy to believe that events which follow one another closely in time are in fact related. Furthermore, although it is quite easy to disprove the existence of this causal relationship, which is often discounted for that reason, there is also the factor which may probably have something to do with lingering superstition, causing individuals to retain the possibility that in some dimly felt way a connection exists.

Time relationship is only one of several dimensional relationships that may be believed to exist in a causal connection. Others may be similarity of subject, the nature of the occurrences, the appearance of some form of justification, just desserts, and so on. But they all have in common the assumption of a causal connection, because causal connections of this nature can and do exist in the normal course of events. A clear case of causal connections produces this kind of relationship between events, but between events this does not necessarily, or even often, imply a causal relationship.

In order to assess why we are so likely to assert connections which in logic cannot really exist, we are bound to seek precipitating or catalytic factors in an area other than in logical thought. I suspect that this area is one that is usually dismissed, but is nevertheless extremely prevalent and potent, the concept of a mystical world of forces which somehow surrounds and totally engulfs that which our senses reveal to us as existing. Yet this mystical world is one which most of us would deny if asked and feel uncomfortable about if pressed to explain. The fact that the world as we know it is wholly the creation of human beings in that it is only knowable by the interpretation of our sense data, means that an actual mystical world is no more unlikely as a form of interpretation than the usual one. Hence it is possible that the strong urge to avoid blame may still contain some element of propitiation.

CONSONANCE AND SELF-JUSTIFICATION

In 1993 two boys, then 10 years old, were found guilty of luring James Bolger, a 2-year-old, away from his mother in a shopping arcade, taking him two and half miles away to a railway, beating him with sticks, stones and an iron bar, throwing paint over him and eventually leaving his battered body on the railway line. When brought to the police station and questioned separately both boys sought to lay the major responsibility for the death of this small boy, hardly more than a baby, onto the other.

Leaving aside what actually motivated the 10-year-olds to perform such an act of intense and deliberate brutality on a small defenceless child, there emerges clearly the basis of the 'rational' aspect of scapegoating, and at the early age of 10. While no doubt lying desperately about their part in the process, the ultimate technique each had already developed was to attempt to diminish his share of blame by trying to increase the share of the other. Where, as in this case, there was no hope of escaping some justified blame, the technique of attempting to readjust the comparative share of responsibility is widespread. Even in such depraved and degraded circumstances as the deliberate abduction and murder of a toddler, it mattered to each of the defendants that his share of the allocated blame and responsibility should be, as far as possible, diminished and the share apportioned to the other comparatively increased.

Psychologists have often discussed the phenomenon of self-justification, the necessity to offer an apparently rational explanation of otherwise inexplicable behaviour which is also compatible with the individual's self-image. Given that the self-image held by most individuals contains a large element of self-regard and belief that they are actually good, then the rationalisation of bad behaviour has to contain either a shift to outside authority, as in the case of Lieutenant Calley and in Milgram's experiments in obedience (1974), or a reduction in size and importance if there is no obvious outside agent to blame.

Cognitive dissonance theory has an attraction as an explanation because of its very simplicity in that it states that to hold two or more dissonant opinions about ourselves and our behaviour concurrently generates a tension, a discomfort, which needs to be discharged or changed so that those opinions can once more be consonant and compatible. The energy that is alleged to stem from the recognition of dissonance is the main power that energises action to adjust the incompatibilities. Essentially the mainspring of action can be seen to arise not so much in the recognition of the incompatibility of feelings, opinions and actions but in the perceived threat to the individual which comes as a consequence of them.

Undoubtedly, as the child psychiatrist maintained in court, the two 10-year-olds had a sufficiently clear idea of the difference between right and wrong actions to know, without equivocation, that what they were doing, and indeed appeared to have planned to do, was wrong. Yet they did not stop. They did not, as far as we know, confess what they had done when they were picked up in the police search. If dissonance between their knowledge of right and wrong and their behaviour had existed it only emerged in terms of their need for each to diminish his share of the blame.

The basic attempt to excuse behaviour, to offer explanation if not to ask for exoneration, appears to be absolutely fundamental, a very deep and basic human response pattern triggered by the perception of threat – not just any threat, but one that is seen as life-threatening or one that is extremely damaging to the self-esteem or even to promise unpleasantness or suffering of a high order.

Under such pressure one apparently promising manoeuvre is to blame someone else. If others were involved, this is a comparatively simple tactic; if they were not, then the alternative may well be to appeal to a lack of rationality which has some standing as an appeal not for exoneration but for understanding.

When we consider substitution as a method of avoiding obloquy either in the case of a charged individual or a group, it is interesting to note that although in most instances the effect is transient and the relief temporary, this may be all that is needed to obtain a respite to set in motion more effective ways of coping with the problem, as we saw in Chapter 9. If, however, it is regarded as a solution, then almost invariably, because the basic causes of the problem remain untackled, the problem will tend to re-emerge unless unforeseen circumstances arise to change those causes and the situation in which they operate. There is, therefore, a very basic need for techniques that expose the process of scapegoating for what it is, a temporary, transient and often very costly method of evading or ignoring the fundamental causes of individual or group distress.

Even the classical form of scapegoating can be seen to be transient. I have argued that the ancients, by virtue of the inherent tendency of human beings to sin, required this to be performed at least annually or even more frequently. So although the sin was eradicated it was also only a transient measure and the basic necessity for its performance, sinning, was left intact. Expiation would continue to be needed.

Thus I believe that it is only possible to assert that scapegoating is a group maintenance technique if it is also recognised that it is a transient or recurring ameliorative which eventually occludes the real causes of the experienced problems. It may well have two main beneficial functions: first, it can give a temporary respite from pressure, which may be all that is needed in some systems for a form of self-readjustment to take place; second, it may give the group enough time to re-examine what is actually happening and to devise different and less hurtful methods of coping, or perhaps to realise that no adjustment is possible.

BELIEF SYSTEM

Most modern words used to describe the process of scapegoating indicate an attitude of contempt for those who become or are forced into the substitute position of victim. They appear to suggest that if people are so unwary, so stupid, so unsophisticated as not to realise that they are being made use of, then that is their misfortune. Truly it is part of the belief that there is one born every minute and they are gullible and there to be taken advantage of, so that the streetwise, the knowing ones can gain advantage or, at the very least, survival.

This attitude has a long history, but it tends to show most clearly in two areas: first, the change from the ritual and mystical element of classical scapegoating to the deliberate and intentional victimisation of the so-called gullible for personal advantage or survival; second, the marked increase in what can be called the individual use of scapegoating rather than its use as a communal cleansing process.

The expectation of punishment, which was so prevalent among the ancients, is no less prevalent today with the major difference that today's punishing agents are the society in which the individual lives and the individual himself. In some sense this might give individuals the idea that society is more fallible than an all-seeing god, so modern scapegoating procedures possess much less of a bargain struck with the punishing agency and infinitely more of a plot to deceive. Thus the communication system, which was such an essential part of the classical scapegoat procedure in opening up the prospect of being able to plead for forgiveness, to offer expiation and to accept penance, is used to obfuscate and hide, to deflect scrutiny away from the culprit onto his or her selected victim.

This in turn leads to another major difference between old and new forms: the public acceptance of fault allied to the means to get rid of it as opposed to the private acceptance of fault and the means to deflect its consequences. In each case survival is at stake, but whereas the former carried with it the essential fact of cleansing, the modern process seems to produce no such effect, merely the desire that guilt shall remain hidden and unexpiated, with the damaging consequences of wrong-doing being meanwhile evaded. The transfer system no longer works in that sense, because there is no longer the belief that it will.

In the case of groups and organisations the symbolic and cathartic nature of scapegoating stands clearly revealed. Where intense frustration exists the energy build up is quite strong, and if this can be discharged in the form of blaming some person or group for its existence then, whether the accusation is true or false, the discharge of discomfort and tension can take place, irritation is reduced and the ability to concentrate, which had been drastically reduced by anxiety, is restored to functional levels. If, as we have seen to be possible, this discharge frees energy, allowing a practical effort to be made to cope with the actual causes of frustration, then the cost to the group, and in particular to the victim, may have been worth while. But all too often the result is regarded as permanent rather than temporary and eventually the frustration reasserts itself unless information and help external to those involved is invoked and a clear attempt is made to deal with the real causes.

MISTAKES

People make mistakes and errors of judgement, and sometimes they indulge intentionally in hurt processes. It is right that these factors should not be hidden, because much of human social behaviour is based upon an appreciation of the levels of trust that are appropriate in given situations. However, it is neither an effective nor a moral method of coping when the mistakes of one individual generate consequences that are expiated by another, unless the other was equally responsible for them.

Injustice and resentment are potent breeders of hostility and aggression, and unless scapegoats are willing victims these factors need to be taken into consideration. Even when willing, scapegoats are individuals who are used; their willingness does not detract from the fact that others are gaining at their expense. One of the prime reasons for choosing a victim who appears powerless is that the resentment and hostility that can be engendered by victimisation stands small chance of being effectively concentrated into revenge by such people. But mistakes of assessment are made, as we have seen, and revenge does occasionally occur, often in a form which actually makes the vengeful scapegoat more likely to produce evident justification for being attacked further.

FINAL ASSESSMENT

The process of scapegoating seems to fall clearly into two main categories: namely, as a rational strategy to deflect opprobrium, censure and possible punishment; and as an irrational move to relieve relatively intolerable pressures emanating from mainly unknown sources. In most cases both processes involve others, frequently largely innocent of complicity, who take upon themselves or have thrust upon them the blame that should rightly be placed elsewhere. The cost to these scapegoated victims is often high; in the past, and not infrequently now, it has meant their deaths. But the essential fact is that in either form of the process, unless exceptional circumstances prevail, the cost to the victim buys only a transient solution. Where the actual causes of distress are unknown, the process can only produce a temporary relief unless the circumstances that are the real cause of the problems change. This is not a likely result of the scapegoating procedure for the simple reason that it is essentially a process of the relatively blind discharge of tensions onto a convenient focus.

The most that can be achieved, therefore, is a temporary cessation of distress, or perhaps diminution would be more accurate. If this is considered to be a totally effective solution then the problem is almost inevitably set to recur, and perhaps the same temporary solution will be applied again. This is the reason for the recorded value of the scapegoat in group literature as the person who is driven to the periphery of the group but seldom wholly driven completely out. If the victim is driven out, then all the evidence tends to point to the group choosing another as soon as tension once more becomes intolerable.

If the temporary lull is regarded as an opportunity free of the strains of tension in which a realistic search for the actual causes of that tension and distress can be made and a more effective method of coping sought, then the process of buying time will have been appropriate. Otherwise the process has to be viewed as one in which peers are sacrificed purely for a temporary solution, and that is a very high price to pay for what often turns out to be very little.

The other form of the scapegoating process most frequently found in public life is a form of confidence trick in which one person, in order to maintain his or her position, cynically offers a substitute to his or her attackers. The only morally sound approach to this must be that of confrontation and exposure of the nature of the attack. In some cases the attack on an individual or group is itself a scapegoating procedure, and where this is so there may well be some mild justification for the attempt to escape from an unwarranted assault by the processes of substitution and deflection.

In this book I have attempted to trace a particular behaviour pattern that was given a title by William Tyndale in 1530 but has been used since that time to describe behaviour which existed hundreds of years before Tyndale's time, and indeed ever since. I have argued that this behaviour pattern springs from a common and extremely durable human motivation which can be relatively crudely described as a compelling need to avoid the hurtful consequences of certain kinds of behaviour. But, as we have seen, the manifestations of this behavioural need are shaped by the belief system of the society in which the process occurs. In effect, the main predisposing factors are the individual and/or society's perception of who or what is the supervising agent. In ancient days the gods fulfilled this role; in current society, although there is still the same strong perception in religious communities, the main perception seems to be that society itself, or at least some fairly well-defined part of it, possesses the power formerly ascribed to the gods.

There is one other fact in this perception of power which seems to bridge, in some obscure way, the difference between gods and the society – i.e there is some evidence that in some circumstances individuals see themselves as supervisory and persecuting agents.

Indeed, the term 'some circumstances' is misleading. It would be truer to say that such self-regulatory and punitive behaviour is ubiquitous, but the degree of the intensity of its application or its rebuttal varies considerably in different situations.

So it is reasonable to assume that the basic urge to avoid hurtful responsibility is as old as human beings, only the manifestations have changed mainly in accord with the changes in society. Thus from the expressly communal activity, religious in the widest sense, of the ancients, the modern equivalent is a great deal more centred around individuals and small groups where the belief system is at least similar and not so diffuse and disparate as in the general body of vast modern societies. The selfish element has also seemingly increased as society has become more oriented towards the independence, however spurious, of the individual.

Indeed the truer descendant of the classical form of scapegoating, so elegantly and succinctly described in Leviticus, must be what I have designated as the rational/deflective form in these pages, not the irrational/transferring form which has become so important since scapegoating lost most of its ritual and mystic significance and society became extremely aware of the processes of unconscious motivation.

Consider the elements. The ancient ritual admittedly founded in a particular form of belief which involved divine beings, was a consciously performed act, the main purpose of which was to deflect punishment for wrong-doing and to seek absolution from beings considered able to give it. The ultimate purpose was a form of cleansing, producing a liberating effect which freed the community to live their lives unhindered by either a burden of guilt or of imminent punishment. A price was paid, often in terms of a scarce commodity, e.g. food, but equally often in terms of human beings, e.g. criminals and outcasts, of little value to society.

The modern public scapegoater pursues a rational cause to deflect imminent punishment, opprobrium, personality assassination onto others. His or her main purpose is to survive; the technique is conscious; the cost, if the ploy is successful, is mainly borne by someone or something other than the focal individual. The outcome is that this individual is absolved of responsibility and, like the ancients, is free to pursue his or her course.

On the other hand, the irrational/transferring form of scapegoating with which most people who work in groups are much more familiar, may appear only to have the essential and basic motivation in common with ancient ritual. Most of the process is neither conscious nor deliberate; it does not seek therefore to deflect opprobrium but to relieve intolerable tension; it is relatively inexplicable as far as the scapegoaters are concerned, but it does have the effect of clearing them and those who support them to move forward if only in a transient and temporary fashion.

However, such an irrational process can have other things in common with the ancient ritual apart from the ubiquitous motivation: first, there is a need for repetition and, second, it is usually a communal or group activity with a communal or group goal as its desired outcome.

As most forms of coping with potentially damaging behaviour are concerned with bringing into consciousness the behaviour itself and also its consequences, the problems of management and resolution of scapegoating are of very different kinds in the two forms of the process. In the conscious and deliberate form the search, if search is applicable, has to be for an alternative form of coping. As the self-preservation theme is essentially very strong, the scapegoating can only truly be resolved by the scapegoater(s) admitting responsibility for the circumstances for which they are or were under attack. As such an admission might well defeat the essential goal of preservation, this is not a likely outcome and the process of discovering evidence and of confrontation becomes the only alternative.

On the other hand, as the transferring process is largely unknown to those who employ it, the process of change involves exposure and the development of different, more conscious and more rational ways of coping. Indeed, as we have seen often enough in this kind of scapegoating, the revelation of the true causes of distress and frustration have resulted in a cessation of the victimisation. The development of the recognition of the causes is then the necessary prelude to creating less hurtful ways of dealing with them and also of reducing the tensions involved. The sacrificial element is still strong here in the sense of the need to 'throw someone to the wolves', so there must still be some residual sense that sacrifice will of itself put things right. The process of scapegoating, however described, will continue to be used as long as human beings are frustrated and brought to a state of tension either by factors they see all too clearly or by factors that have no discernible source.

The last word in this context can safely be left to Huckleberry Finn, who said:

That's just the way; a person does a low-down thing, and then he don't want to take no consequences of it. Thinks as long as he can hide it, it ain't no disgrace.

(Twain 1975: 207)

Bibliography

Adorno, T., Frenkel-Brunswick, E., Levinson, D.J. and Sandford, R.N. (1950) *The Authoritarian Personality*, Harper & Row: New York.

Alexander, F. (1948) 'Development of the ego psychology', in S. Lorand (ed.) *Psycho Analysis Today*, George Allen & Unwin: London.

Argyle, M. (1976) *Social Interaction*, Tavistock Publications: London.

Aronson, E. (1980) *The Social Animal* (3rd edition) Freeman & Co.: San Francisco.

Aveline, M. and Dryden, W. (eds) (1988) *Group Therapy in Britain*, Open University Press: Milton Keynes.

Baigent, M., Leigh, R. and Lincoln, H. (1986) *The Messianic Legacy*, Guild Publishing: London.

Bates, B. (1983) *The Way of Wyrd*, Century Publishing: London.

Bell, N.W. and Vogel, E.F. (1970) 'The emotionally disturbed child as the family scapegoat', in T.M. Mills and S. Rosenberg (eds) *Readings in the Sociology of Small Groups*, Prentice-Hall: Englewood Cliffs, N.J.

Berkovitz, I.H. (1972) *Adolescents Grow in Groups*, Brunner/Mazel: New York.

Berkowitz, L. and Green, J.A. (1965) 'The stimulus qualities of the scapegoat' in A. Yates (ed.) *Frustration and Conflict*, Van Nostrand: New York.

Brewer, E.C. (1978) *Dictionary of Phrase and Fable*, Book Club Associates: London.

Brown, D. and Pedder, J. (1979) *Introduction to Psychotherapy*, Tavistock Publications: London.

Button, L. (1974) *Development Work with Adolescents*, University of London Press.

Campbell, J. (1973) *Myths to Live By*, Souvenir Press (Educational & Academic): London.

Caplan, G. (1964) *Principles of Preventive Psychiatry*, Tavistock Publications: London.

Clark, K. (1971) *Civilisation: A Personal View*, BBC & John Murray: London.

Coch, L. and French, J.R.P. (1948) 'Overcoming resistance to change', *Human Relations* 1: 512–32.

Cowger, C.D. (1979) 'Conflict and conflict management', *Working with Groups* **2**(4), Haworth Press: New York.

Cuppitt, D. (1985) *The Sea of Faith*, BBC: London.

Davis, J.H. (1969) *Group Performance*, Addison-Wesley: Reading, Mass.

Dentler, R.A. and Erikson, K.T. (1970) 'The function of deviance in groups', in T.M. Mills and S. Rosenberg (eds) *Readings in the Sociology of Small Groups*, Prentice-Hall: Englewood Cliffs, N.J.

Dollard, J., Miller, N.E., Dobb, L.W., Mowrer, O.H. and Sears, R.R. (1939) *Frustration & Aggression*, Yale University Press: New Haven.

Douglas, T. (1983) *Groups; Understanding People Gathered Together*, Tavistock Publications: London.

Drever, J. (1952) *Dictionary of Psychology*, Penguin Books: Harmondsworth.

Eban, Abba (1984) *Heritage: Civilisation and the Jews*, Weidenfeld & Nicolson: London.

Feldman, R.A. (1969) 'Group integration: intense interpersonal dislike and social groupwork intervention', *Social Work(US)* **14**(3): 30–9.

Feldman, R.A. and Wodarski, J.S. (1975) *Contemporary Approaches to Group Treatment*, Jossey-Bass: London.

Foulkes, S.H. and Anthony, E.J. (1957) *Group Psychotherapy*, Penguin Books: Harmondsworth.

Frazer, J. (1978) *The Illustrated Golden Bough*, Mary Douglas (ed.), Book Club Associates: London.

French, J.R.P. and Raven, B. (1959) 'The bases of social power', in M.D. Cartwright (ed.) *Studies in Social Power*, Institute for Social Research, University of Michigan: Ann Arbor.

Frey, D.E. (1979) 'Understanding and managing conflict', in S. Eisenberg and L.E. Patterson (eds) *Helping Clients with Special Concerns*, Rand McNally: Chicago.

Garland, J.A. and Kolodny, R.L. (1966) 'Characteristics and resolution of scapegoating', in S. Bernstein (ed.) *Explorations in Groupwork*, National Conference of Social Workers.

Garvin, C.D. (1981) *Contemporary Groupwork*, Prentice-Hall: Englewood Cliffs, N.J.

Gascoigne, B. (1980) *The Christians*, Granada Publishing: London.

Geen, R.G. (1972) *Aggression*, General Learning Press (module): Morristown, NJ.

Gilbert, W.S. (1885) *The Mikado*.

Goffman, C. (1969) *Presentation of Self in Everyday Life*, Penguin Books: Harmondsworth.

Graves, R. (1961) *The White Goddess*, Faber & Faber: London.

Green, M. (1988) *The Gods of the Celts*, Allan Sutton: Stroud.

Hawkins, P. (1979) 'Staff learning in therapeutic communities; the relationship of supervision to self-learning' in R.D. Hinshelwood and N. Manning (eds) *Therapeutic Communities*, Routledge & Kegan Paul: London.

Heap, K. (1964) 'The scapegoat role in youth groups', *Case Conference* 215–21.

—— (1977) *Group Theory for Social Workers: An Introduction*, Pergamon Press: Oxford.

—— (1985) *The Practice of Social Work with Groups: a Systematic Approach*, George Allen & Unwin: London.

Heider, F. (1958) 'Social perception and phenomenal causality', in R. Taguiri and L. Petrullo (eds) *Person, Perception and Interpersonal Behaviour*, Stanford University Press: California.

Hinksman, B. (1988) 'Gestalt Group Therapy', in M. Aveline and W. Dryden (eds) *Group Therapy in Britain*, Open University Press: Milton Keynes, pp. 65–87.

Hinshelwood, R.D. (1979) 'Supervision as an exchange system', in R.D. Hinshelwood and N. Manning (eds) *Therapeutic Communities*, Routledge & Kegan Paul: London.

Johnson, H.M. (1961) *Sociology: A Systematic Introduction*, Routledge & Kegan Paul: London.

Jones, E.E. and Nisbett, R.E. (1971) *The Actor and the Observer: Divergent Perceptions of the Causes of Behaviour*, General Learning Press (module): Morristown, NJ.

Kelman, H.C. and Lawrence, L.H. (1972) 'Assignment of responsibility in the case of Lt. Calley: preliminary report on a national survey', *Journal of Social Issues* **228**(1): 177–212.

Kennard, D. (1988) 'The therapeutic community', in M. Aveline and W. Dryden (eds) *Group Therapy in Britain*, Open University Press: Milton Keynes, pp. 153–84.

Kenny, M. (1993) 'In a violent world, parents should be last to be blamed', *Daily Telegraph* 17 February: 18.

Kepner, E. (1980) 'Gestalt group process', in B. Feder and R. Ronall (eds) *Beyond the Hot Seat*, Brunner/Mazel: New York.

King, F. (1975) *Magic: The Western Tradition*, Book Club Associates: London.

Konopka, G. (1963) *Social Group Work*, Prentice-Hall: Englewood Cliffs, N.J.

Koran (1990) *The Koran*, translated by N.J. Dawood, Penguin Books: Harmondsworth.

Kramer, H. and Sprenger, J. (1971) *Malleus Maleficorum (1486)*, translated by Montague Summers, Arrow Books: London.

Kraupl-Taylor, F.K. (1964) 'The uses of scapegoats', *New Society* 9 January.

Kraupl-Taylor, F.K. and Rey, J.H. (1953) 'The scapegoat motif in society and its manifestations in a therapeutic group', *International Journal of Psychoanalysis* **34**: 253–64.

Leach, M. (ed.) (1950) *Standard Dictionary of Folklore, Mythology & Legend*, Funk & Wagnalls: New York.

Leslie, M. (1991) 'The unsung saviours', *Daily Telegraph* 6 June: 9.

Liddell, H.G. and Scott, R. (1896) *Lexicon*, Clarendon Press: Oxford.

Long, S. (1992) *A Structural Analysis of Small Groups*, Routledge: London.

MacLennan, B.W. and Felsenfeld, N. (1968) *Group Counselling & Psychotherapy with Adolescents*, Columbia University Press: New York.

Maddox, B. (1993) 'Why television is not the real culprit', *Daily Telegraph* 24 March: 16.

Mann, R.D. (1967) *Interpersonal Styles & Group Development*, Wiley: New York.

Mauriac, F. (1961) *Child Martyrs (Second Thoughts)*. [Publisher unknown.]

Medcof, J. and Roth, J. (eds) (1979) *Approaches to Psychology*, Open University Press: Milton Keynes.

Milgram, S. (1974) *Obedience to Authority*, Harper & Row: New York.

Napier, R.N. and Gershenfeld, M.K. (1973) *Groups: Theory & Experience*, Houghton Mifflin: Boston.

Nicholson, J. (1977) *Habits*, Macmillan: London.

Northen, H. (1969) *Social Work with Groups*, Columbia University Press: New York.

Opie, I. and Opie, P. (1959) *The Language and Lore of Schoolchildren*, Oxford University Press: Oxford.

Pegg, B. (1981) *Rites & Riots: Folk Customs of Britain & Europe*, Blandford Press: UK.

Price, C. (1991) 'Scapegoats of justice', *The Guardian* 11 June: 19.

Raven, B.H. and Rubin, J.Z. (1976) *Social Psychology: People in Groups*, Wiley: New York.

Renault, M. (1979) *The Praise Singer*, Book Club Associates: London.

Russell, W.M.S. (1964) 'Aggression: new light from animals', *New Society* 10 February: 13–14.

Ryecroft, C. (1972) *A Critical Dictionary of Psychoanalysis*, Penguin Books: Harmondsworth.

Schofield, M. (1971) *The Strange Case of Pot*, Penguin Books: Harmondsworth.

Sherif, C.W. (1976) *Orientation in Social Psychology*, Harper & Row: New York.

Shulman, L. (1968) 'Scapegoats, group workers and pre-emptive intervention', *Social Work (US)* **12**(2): 37–43.

Simon, E. (1967) *The Reformation*, Time Life International (Nederland) NV.

Skynner, A.C.R. (1971a) 'Indications for and against conjoint family therapy', *Social Work Today* 1 July.

—— (1971b) 'A group analytic approach to conjoint family therapy', *Social Work Today* 15 July.

—— (1971c) 'The minimum sufficient network', *Social Work Today* 29 July.

Storr, A. (1968) *Human Aggression*, Allen Lane, Penguin Press: UK.

Tolstoy, N. (1985) *The Quest for Merlin*, Hamish Hamilton: London.

Twain, M. (1953) *The Adventures of Huckleberry Finn*, Puffin Books, Penguin Books: Harmondsworth, p. 207.

Whiffen, R. (1978) 'Family therapy: the family group as the medium for change', in N. McCaughan (ed.) *Group Work: Learning & Practice*, George Allen & Unwin: London.

Wilden, A. (1980) *System & Structure* (2nd edition), Tavistock Publications: London.

Index